Decision Making in Paramedic Practice

CANADIAN EDITION

Edited by Andy Collen and Sean Teed

Printing history
First UK edition published in 2015. Reprinted 2015, 2016, 2017, 2019.
Second UK edition published 2022.
Third edition first published 2024.
This first Canadian edition first published 2026. Reprinted via print on demand from 2026.

The authors and publisher welcome feedback from the users of this book.
Please contact the publisher:
Class Professional Media Canada Inc., registered at 2345 Yonge Street, Suite 300, Toronto, Ontario, M4P 2E5
Telephone: +441278 472 800
Email: info@class.co.uk
Website: www.classprofessional.ca
Class Professional Media Canada Inc. is a subsidiary of Class Publishing Ltd, registered at The Exchange, Express Park, Bristol Road, Bridgwater TA6 4RR, United Kingdom
A CIP catalogue record for this book is available from the British Library

Paperback ISBN: 9781801612180
ePub ISBN: 9781801612203
ePDF ISBN: 9781801612197
Cover design by Nicky Borowiec
Designed and typeset by S4Carlisle Publishing Services
Printed in the UK by Hobbs

This book is printed on paper from responsible sources. Refer to local recycling guidance on disposal of this book.

Contents

Land Acknowledgement ix

About the Authors xi

Preface xv

Introduction – *Who Is This Book For?* xvii

1: Paramedic Practice: The Ongoing Journey of Paramedic Evolution 1
Sean Teed, Andy Collen and Si Robinson

A Historical Glimpse 1

Advocacy 3

Legislation and Regulation 4

The Evolving Role of Paramedics and Changing Practice Settings 6

Patient Demography and Epidemiology 8

Conclusion 12

Reflective Exercises 13

2: Professional and Ethical Issues 15
Si Robinson and Andy Collen

Introduction 15

Professional Regulation and Standards 17

Scope of Practice: Individual Skills, Speciality or Organizational Policy? 18

Fitness to Practise and Sanctions 19

Professional Identity 20

Autonomy 22

Summarizing the Notion of Professional Identity 25

Decision Making Through the Lens of Bioethics 26

A Brief Overview of Bioethics 27

Ethical Decision Making in Paramedic Practice 31

Moving Towards a Paramedic Ethical Model 39

Patient-centred Care 42

Confidentiality: The Crossroads Between Professionalism and Bioethics 43

	Competence and Confidence in Practice	**44**
	Professional Insight	**45**
	Conclusion	**46**
	Reflective Exercises	**47**
	Further Reading	**47**
3:	**Decision-making Theory: Dilemmas and Conundrums** *Si Robinson and Andy Collen*	**49**
	Introduction	**49**
	Models of Reasoning	**51**
	Deductive Reasoning	**51**
	Inductive Reasoning	**52**
	Abductive Reasoning	**53**
	Causal Reasoning	**54**
	The Hypothetico-deductive Model	**55**
	Heuristics – Pattern Recognition	**56**
	Dual Process Theory	**58**
	Naturalistic Decision Making	**60**
	The Cognitive Continuum	**61**
	Patient Safety: Error, Blame and Just Culture	**61**
	System Safety and Reliability	**63**
	The Nature of Errors, Mistakes and Violations	**64**
	Blame and Moving Towards a Just Culture	**67**
	Checklists and Structured Communication	**69**
	Human Fallibility and Biased Thinking – Learn Before You Make Mistakes	**70**
	Anchoring	**71**
	Availability	**72**
	Conjunction Bias	**72**
	Optimism and Loss Aversion	**73**
	Other Relevant Biases and Fallacies	**74**
	Conclusion	**78**
	Reflective Exercises	**79**
4:	**Inclusive Decision Making** *Sean Teed, Robert Bonspiel, Bo Escritt, Agatha Nortley-Meshe and Alison Walker,*	**81**
	Why Should We Be Aware of Equality, Diversity and Inclusion?	**81**

Health and Wellness: A New Guiding Principle 81
Why is Positionality Important? 84
What Is Bias and Why Does It Happen? 84
In-groups and Out-groups 85
System-1 and System-2 Thinking 85
Unconscious Bias 86
Conscious Bias 86
How Can Bias Impact Decision Making? 87
How Can Paramedics Consider and Mitigate Against Bias Within Their Roles? 87
Identifying Unconscious Bias 87
Unconscious Bias Training 88
Being an Ally 88
Moving from Cultural Competency to Cultural Humility 90
Psychological Safety 91
Metacognition 92
Slowing Down the Thought Process 92
Two Brains Are Better Than One 92
Intentionally Diversify Your Network 93
Reciprocal Mentoring 93
Communication Skills 94
The Elements of Communication 94
Verbal Communication 95
Language and Vocabulary 95
The Importance of Communication with Each Other 97
Written Communication 97
Social and Cultural Context 98
Challenges to Communication 98
Improving Communication Awareness 98
Culture and Ethnicity: The Impact on Disease Manifestations and Effect on Health Outcomes 100
Conclusion 104
Reflective Exercises 104

5: The Evolution of the Paramedic as a Critical Thinker 107
Andy Collen

Critical Thinking in Everyday Life and Paramedic Practice 108
Values-based Decision Making and Healthcare Practice 110

Information Processing 113

Barriers to Critical Thinking 117

Egotism *vs* Humility 120

Selfishness: Emotional Influence and Personal Values 122

Intuition and Experience in Critical Thinking 125

Decision Point Management: Taking Control at Each Stage 126

Summing Up: Moving from 'What' to 'Why' 130

Conclusion 130

Reflective Exercises 131

Further Resources 131

6: The Garden Gate Test: Putting Decision-making Theory into Practice 133
Andy Collen and Si Robinson

Introduction 133

Defining the Cognitive Continuum 134

Experience and Competence 136

Judgement and Sense-making 141

Conclusion 145

Reflective Exercises 146

7: Refining and Improving the Application of Decision Making in Practice 147
Kieren Pugh and Andy Collen

Introduction 147

Consolidating Your Own Experience 149

Pre- and Post-test Probability 150

Over-testing 151

Feedback 152

Considering Professional Risk and Consequence 154

Mitigating Risk: Management *vs* Avoidance 154

Documentation 154

Practising Defensibly, Rather Than Defensively 157

Considering Sinister Presentations 158

Working Together for Your Patient 159

Collaborative Decision Making 159

Reasonable Decisions in Practice 162

Approaching Professional Conflict and Encouraging Challenge 163

Balancing Thoroughness and Effectiveness with the Needs of the Wider Population 163

Conclusion 165

Reflective Exercises 166

8: Case-based Discussion (Case Studies, Reflection, Action Learning) 167

Andy Collen, Si Robinson, Kieren Pugh and Sean Teed

Introduction 167

Case Study 1: 32-year-old Female with a Headache 168

Case Study 2: 45-year-old Male with Productive Cough and Chest Pain 172

Case Study 3: 78-year-old Female Fallen with a Minor Head Injury and Taking Anticoagulant Therapy 176

Case Study 4: 29-year-old Female with Respiratory Illness 180

Case Study 5: 36-year-old Female with Abdominal Pain 185

Case Study 6: 23-year-old Female Car Crash 189

Case Study 7: 40-year-old Male with GI Bleed 192

Appendix 197

Glossary 199

Bibliography 205

Index 221

Land Acknowledgement

The authors and editors of this book acknowledge that this work has been adapted for use in the Traditional Territories and homelands of First Nations peoples, Métis, and Inuit in what we now call Canada. We respect the histories, languages, and cultures of Indigenous peoples that enrich our communities. We also recognize that actions and inactions have had a negative impact on the health and wellness of Indigenous peoples. In the spirit of reconciliation, we aim to address these wrongs in our principles and improve our role and actions by incorporating knowledge and understanding into our practices in partnership with Indigenous communities.

About the Authors

Andy Collen
DipHE MSc DipUMC FCPara
Andy is currently a Consultant Paramedic at South East Coast Ambulance Service, co-leading on the Trust's urgent care specialist/advanced paramedic practice programmes, professional standards and scope of practice. He has recently finished a secondment at the Healthcare Safety Investigation Branch as a National Investigator. Andy is also a Clinical Ambassador at the Clinical Human Factors Group.

Andy was the Medicines and Prescribing Project Lead for the College of Paramedics, having worked alongside NHS England on independent prescribing for advanced paramedics, as well as other projects, such as the review of paramedic medicines exemptions. He has contributed to the College's published documents relating to medicines, and has prepared Practice Guidance for Prescribers, Implementation Guidance for Prescribing and Practice Guidance for Exemptions.

Andy has written and contributed to several publications relating to paramedic practice, such as *Decision Making in Paramedic Practice*, and is a visiting senior lecturer at the University of Surrey.

Sean Teed
MEd, BAppB:ES, Critical Care Paramedic
Sean currently works as a licensed paramedic in the province of Nova Scotia, Canada and is also an interprofessional educator and instructor at Dalhousie University. He facilitates and co-facilitates medical students within the faculty of medicine and learners within the physician assistant program. Sean has practice experience in ground transport and flight paramedicine, emergency department practice and within the ground ambulance and paramedic system(s) in Ontario and Nova Scotia.

Sean has developed curriculum for all licensure and practice levels of paramedic and the Emergency Medical Responder. He was the inaugural elected council member to the College of Paramedics Nova Scotia (now the Nova Scotia Regulator of Paramedicine). Sean participated in the development of the Paramedic Essential Regulatory Requirements with the Canadian Organization of Paramedic Regulators and contributed to the development of the Paramedic Association of Canada's National Competency Framework Paramedics as an emergency department subject matter expert working group lead.

Sean's personal vision is to put care back in career and since the completion of his masters, challenges the historical approaches to paramedic education program delivery to be more inclusive and socially responsive. Sean lives close to Peggy's Cove in Nova Scotia with his wife and family and enjoys life by the salt water.

Robert Bonspiel

Robert Bonspiel is the Paramedic Chief and General Director of First Nations Paramedics, the only Indigenous-owned and operated, provincially contracted ambulance service in Québec, Canada. A federal and provincial lobbyist, he has testified before two provincial commissions on Indigenous–government relations in emergency medical services.

He serves as the sole Indigenous and Québec representative on the Board of Directors of the Canadian Paramedic Memorial Foundation. He is currently advising Québec's Ministry of Health and Ministry of Education, as well as provincial CEGEPs, on Indigenous-led pathways to increase the representation of Indigenous paramedics within their own communities. In parallel, he is working with provincial partners to implement culturally grounded, community-integrated care models that complement local health centres and existing first responder frameworks.

He brings over three decades of experience as a paramedic in First Nations communities, alongside 18 years as a First Nations police officer across Québec. His perspectives on developing culturally grounded, Indigenous-inclusive EMS models have been featured in EMS publications, and he is a recipient of the King Charles III Coronation Medal.

Bo Escritt

Honorary Fellow of the College of Paramedics FCIPD FIEDP

Bo works as an Equality, Diversity and Inclusion (EDI) professional and has worked with both the Association of Ambulance Chief Executives (AACE) and the College of Paramedics to support their work on the advancement of the EDI agenda working on race, disability, gender, sexual orientation and social-economic background. She currently works part time as Head of EDI for an NHS trust; alongside this role Bo works as an EDI consultant providing strategic direction and training to several organizations.

Bo is an Honorary Fellow of the College of Paramedics and a Fellow of the Chartered Institute of Personnel and Development. Her career spans the private, charity and public sector, including a number of years working for Amnesty International and several years working with various trusts within the NHS.

Bo holds a diploma in coaching from Cambridge University and is a fully accredited executive and life coach as well as a mentor. She is also a Fellow of the Institute of Equality and Diversity Professionals.

Bo is an advocate for social justice, equity and a fairer opportunity for all. She feels privileged to have a career in which her purpose, passion and values are aligned.

Agatha Nortley-Meshe

Dr Agatha Nortley-Meshe is a South London GP and the London Regional Medical Director for Primary Care at NHS England.

Agatha has worked across multiple healthcare settings and previously held leadership roles in both commissioning and provider organizations including Croydon CCG and London Ambulance Service. She has a wealth of experience in clinical leadership, clinical governance and service redesign, and has worked on a variety of national, regional and local projects.

Her experiences as a clinical leader and frontline clinician in primary care (in and out of hours), community, urgent and emergency care, 111 and 999 have enabled her to develop a whole system view around healthcare delivery in London, with a unique insight into the interface between primary and urgent care. In addition to this, her extensive experience in healthcare leadership has provided her with a clear understanding of the of social and cultural determinants of health as well as the impact of bias in healthcare delivery and inequity in access and treatment. She is passionate about addressing health inequalities to ensure the best outcomes for patients.

Agatha is an accredited WRES expert and has used this experience to champion the race equality agenda. She is passionate about supporting others to develop confidence and leadership skills and over the years, she has provided informal coaching and mentoring to support personal and career development for healthcare colleagues. In addition to this, from 2011–2016 she provided mentoring to women from several different countries via the Cherie Blair Foundation for Women. She is an online Tutor for the University of London Global MBA Quality Improvement Module and a co-director of DAPS Global – an organization that specializing in leadership, patient safety and Quality Improvement training for frontline and junior clinical staff. She has delivered training workshops and seminars nationally and globally on Quality Improvement, Patient Safety and Racial Equality.

Kieren Pugh
BSc (hons), MSc, DIMC (RCSEd), MCPara

Kieren Pugh works as a Critical Care Paramedic at South East Coast Ambulance Service. He has completed the Diploma in Immediate Medical Care (DIMC) from the Royal College of Surgeons in Edinburgh and has an MSc in Healthcare Practice (Pre-hospital Critical Care) from St George's University of London. Kieren was also involved in publishing a paper in the *Journal of Paramedic Practice* on proning during the coronavirus pandemic. His professional interests include resuscitation and crew resource management.

Si Robinson
MSc DFSEM(UK) MCPara

Si works as a Paramedic Practitioner and MDT Manager for Ringmead Medical Group in Berkshire. His main interests are paediatrics and child health, musculoskeletal medicine and cancer care. He is currently working towards a PhD at the University of Hertfordshire that explores the decision-making relationships of paramedics on ambulances and families of acutely unwell children. He was awarded the Diploma in Musculoskeletal Medicine jointly from the Primary Care Rheumatology and Musculoskeletal Medicine Society and Faculty of Sports and Exercise Medicine (to which he sits as a member and diplomate member respectively).

Si also adheres to the Macmillan competency framework for Allied Health Professionals and continues to collaborate with colleagues from Thames Valley Cancer Alliance, Wessex Cancer Alliance and Frimley Park Hospital in improving cancer services.

Si is a member of the College of Paramedics Public Health Specialist Interest Group. Outside of Paramedic Practice, he continues to be a musician, having studied a Master in Performance Science at the Royal College of Music, and is a keen advocate on the positive impact music has on everyone's mental health and wellbeing. He is a Trustee of the Blue Light Symphony Orchestra, a music therapy mental health charity for emergency service personnel. His published works are available here: https://orcid.org/0000-0002-2780-2834

Alison Walker
Alison is the West Midlands Ambulance Service (WMAS) Medical Director and has worked in the NHS for over 35 years. She has been a Consultant in Emergency Medicine for over 20 years and is the National Ambulance Service Medical Director lead on the Royal College of Emergency Medicine (RCEM) Prehospital Emergency Medicine Professional Advisory Group. She has been a prehospital clinician and involved in prehospital education since 1996.

She has also been a member of the JRCALC (Joint Royal Colleges Ambulance Liaison Committee) national committee since 2005, has led on several JRCALC guidelines including on mental health, Acute Behavioural Disturbance and led workstreams on reducing inequalities in care. She Became the JRCALC Chair in January 2020 and is a member of the UK Trauma and Audit Research Network Committee (TARN).

She is an examiner for the Fellowship and Diploma examinations for the Faculty of Prehospital Care of the Royal College of Surgeons of Edinburgh. She has a regional National Institute of Clinical Research network lead role in Trauma and Emergency Care and has authored several journal publications on ambulance service clinical care and clinical pathways and other prehospital topics.

She has interests in prehospital research and improving clinical care.

Preface

Sean Teed

My experience and learning suggest that we ought to encourage folks to reflect on the Calls to Action (2015) and their meaning to us as individuals. This personal acknowledgement is a reflection that I choose to share with you:

Personal Acknowledgement: I am thankful for our families, health, communities, and that we live with nature. I recognize that I was born into privilege and am committed to using this privilege to share knowledge and take action related to Truth and Reconciliation.

Previous editions of this book have done an incredible job at shedding much light on the topic of decision making within the practice of paramedicine! Many theoretical models are presented and well explained with graphics, evidence and cases that are directly relatable to any context of paramedic practice. I am humbled, honoured and excited to have been invited to contribute as an editor to this exceptional work! This team is also excited to be providing an edition that incorporates a Canadian lens – thank you for creating this space!

This edition still includes those models and theories from previous editions, with the goal of beginning to provide some Canadian context to our readers. We will provide a brief history of advocacy and regulatory standards development within Canadian paramedic practice. For decades now, we have supported that health, wellness and healing should take place within the bricks and mortar of a clean environment, free from the dirt and earth provided by nature. This may or may not have impacted our understanding or misunderstanding of how important being in nature can contribute to one's wellbeing. As such, colonialism comes up when reflecting on interpretations of things that are true. Keep this in mind as we continue to be better decision makers.

Chapter 4, 'Inclusive Decision Making', is expanded to provide space for positionality and how positionality impacts one's decision making. Positionality begins to form people's biases and interpretations of life around them and the lens through which they may feel things to be true (Sensoy and DiAngelo, 2017). It is important to be able to value the lens through which we 'see' or interpret the world around us and our experience within it; for it is at this point where we can sincerely begin to have conversations about health and health equity.

Since the completion of my master's in education, I have been privy to both a behind the scenes look at the development of (paramedic) curriculum and how this curriculum informs the decisions that are made for care provided by paramedics. Likewise, as an interprofessional educator and skills instructor at Dalhousie

University in Halifax Nova Scotia, it is interesting to unpack decisions made by medical students and physician assistants going through their initial education.

Simulation for learning (not evaluation), lived experiences, and concepts such as epistemology and positionality begin to provide a brave space for learners to build their decision-making ability. The links between curriculum design and decision making are intriguing and very impactful, resulting in a need to get it right. There are opportunities for health professionals to practice decision making during initial education. However, we need to be diligent in the design of these educational experiences and have expert facilitation unpack these decisions made in the learning environment to ensure the learning translates appropriately to the paramedic practice environment. Most importantly, how it translates to patients and families.

I recognize that I have been privileged to be involved in the contributions to this edition. I value previous contributions by the authors and editors before me. As a lifelong learner, I read through previous editions of this book and gained insight into my own decision-making. We hope that readers at any stage in their career or life will read through this book and begin or continue to reflect on what biases, interpretations and theoretical frameworks will factor into their decision making.

Let's make a decision to put *care back in career*. Care well!

Sean Teed
April 2026

References

Sensoy, O., and DiAngelo, R., (2017). Is everyone really equal 2nd Edition. Teachers College Press

Truth and Reconciliation Commission of Canada: Calls to Action. (2015). Winnipeg, Manitoba.

Introduction
Who Is This Book For?

Andy Collen and Sean Teed

Decision making in paramedicine has increasing levels of complexity for the practitioner here in Canada. Notwithstanding the variability in care expectations from province to province, whether you are ensuring that you are making decisions that align with the ALS-PCS in Ontario or considering the Clinical Practice Guidelines in Nova Scotia, the ongoing and feverish evolution of paramedicine in Canada complicates decision making. As you read this book, you will also consider what you have been taught (or not taught) at entry-to-practice or within continuing professional development learning. Additionally, the reference tools you choose, or which are chosen for you, regarding paramedic practice, where, and how you have been educated all factor into and add to the complexity of sound decision making.

This book is not intended to replace any of the vast amount of evidence and research that exists on decision making. We encourage you to still engage in the evidence that speaks to you in the science and literature relating to decision making. The truly unique aspect of this reading is that there is an intentional goal to include a very specific paramedic lens. In this edition, we are excited to include contributors from within Canada in an attempt to increase the reach of this content.

It is hoped that all paramedics across their career span can benefit from this edition of the book, from diploma and undergraduate paramedic students through to those in advanced practice roles, and all points in between. This book brings together many elements of safe and sound decision making as an autonomous professional. Paramedics, by their very nature, vary in learning styles, and the intention therefore is not to ground the book in any particular practice setting or level of practice. While some examples focus on a particular application of paramedic practice, the reader will be able to apply these to their own personal or professional context.

The original publication of this book was so up-to-date that very little has changed in this Canadian edition. In this edition, we try and introduce the idea of positionality and how this begins to inform our biases and interpretation of what we believe to be true. This edition attempts to include cases and context focused on paramedic practice in Canada. It has been a very deliberate decision to continue to make this edition as accessible as possible, avoiding highly technical language, preferring instead to direct the reader in a way that is readable at first pass, and which informs sufficiently and/or prompts further reading where needed. Importantly, some of the same themes and concepts are covered from different perspectives in some chapters by the various authors, and readers are encouraged to reflect on the nuances presented and not overlook any of the same topics discussed in other parts of the book. Throughout this text, the term 'patient' is used when discussing clinical scenarios in paramedic practice. Readers should note, however, that regulatory language is evolving within Canadian paramedicine and 'client' is increasingly being adopted in alignment with the Canadian Organization of Paramedic Regulators (COPR).

This edition continues to bring together the views, expertise and experience of a range of authors from within paramedic practice or its immediate orbits. Moving from a book with one voice to a new edition that has a range of voices and emphases will, we hope, make the book richer and more informative.

Underscoring the importance of inclusive decision making and the relevance of positionality when making decisions, a small format change is presented in this edition. 'Inclusive Decision Making' is presented as the third chapter and moved up earlier in the reading. Recognizing the international nature of paramedic practice and the importance of cultural awareness and personal choice for patients, it was felt that adding content that allows the reader to reflect on ways to make the care they provide more personal, and which respects the diverse nature of patients, would be beneficial.

The book has eight chapters, which look at a range of theories and concepts based on the role of the paramedic and considering the vast range of challenges that healthcare provides.

1. The book opens by discussing how the paramedic profession and the scope of their decisions have evolved in the Canada. Paramedics have moved from handling mainly high-acuity, low-complexity cases to dealing with a broader range of patients, which also increasingly includes complex, lower-acuity cases. This shift has required paramedics to become more autonomous and adopt a truly holistic approach to patient care and decision-making.
2. The next chapter builds on this to explain in more detail the important aspects of professional regulation and standards in the context of paramedic practice. It highlights the significance of understanding various factors and considerations that guide and regulate the practice of paramedics, ensuring that decisions and care are aligned with established standards, ethics, laws, evidence-based guidance and patient-centred principles.
3. After providing an overview of the background of paramedic practice in the context of decision making, the book moves forward to explain the different theories and models of reasoning and decision making that are commonly used in healthcare, particularly in the context of paramedic practice. Theories include hypothetico-deduction along with other models that allow judgement to build based on consolidated experience in practice.
4. Building on the idea of a paramedic being a responsible critical thinker, the next chapter explores the importance of equality, diversity and inclusion in the context of diagnosis and decision making. This chapter shows how important it is to be conscious of our own biases as healthcare professionals.

5. 'The Evolution of the Paramedic as a Critical Thinker' underscores the significance of critical thinking in healthcare decision making, the need to challenge assumptions and the importance of evidence-based practices. It encourages paramedics to adopt a dynamic and iterative approach to decision making that considers the evolving evidence base.
6. The 'Garden Gate Test' introduces the concept of challenging oneself to ensure confident and optimal decision making in healthcare. It delves into the complexities of balancing knowledge and experience while under pressure and cautioning against overconfidence and the need for a balanced approach. It discusses how decisions in healthcare can have multiple pathways and emphasizes the importance of judgment in making the right decision.
7. Finally, the book ends with a chapter devoted to effective decision-making strategies for paramedics to ensure patient safety and mitigate errors. Topics include a range of real-world type scenarios that cover the kinds of presentations common in many paramedic practice settings.
8. The book wraps up with a number of case studies for you to test your overall understanding of the book as a whole.

Chapter 1

Paramedic Practice: The Ongoing Journey of Paramedic Evolution

Sean Teed, Andy Collen and Si Robinson

Chapter Objectives

This chapter will cover:

- A historical glimpse
- Advocacy
- Legislation and regulation
- Acuity and complexity
- The evolving role of the paramedic.

A Historical Glimpse

The term paramedic was not commonly used until the late 1990s in Canada with much variation in the title and meaning. For example in 1997 the Ministry of Health in Ontario recognized a name change from Ambulance Officer/EMCA to the existing name of 'Paramedic' (PPAO, 2026). Prior to this, 'ambulance driver' was often the term used to identify individuals that worked on ambulances providing care to the sick and injured outside of the bricks and mortar of the hospital. Depending on the province you worked, one would usually work for an ambulance service or within emergency medical services (EMS); and as such you could be certified as an emergency medical attendant, emergency medical care attendant or an ambulance driver, but rarely as a paramedic.

The expectation in early ambulance work was predicated on rapid assessment followed by minimizing on scene time and rapid transport to a hospital for treatment. To work on an ambulance the minimum job requirements were a valid first aid certificate, a class of driver's license that allowed you to drive an ambulance and usually had to pass a street knowledge test. Many ambulance services were operated from funeral homes, born from the ability to transport an individual, living or not, while lying flat. This variation in title and meaning also spilled over into the patient care standards and equipment used to care for the sick and injured on the streets. As many ambulance services were privately owned and operated, standardized equipment was limited (Geddes, Stewart and Baskett, 2017). The typical equipment found on an ambulance, a defibrillator with a built-in cassette tape, an oxygen tank with various masks and a jet ventilator, shovels and body removal bags.

If ambulance services were lucky, they may have been associated with a physician that was interested in providing some form of guidance for the review of cardiac arrest cases. If we consider the historical evolution for paramedicine within Canada, it *may* have been that some of these physicians acted as a catalyst (or mentors) for the evolution of paramedic practice. For instance, physicians like Dr Justin Maloney who advocated for the use of 911 and defibrillation pre-hospitably (University of Ottawa, 2026) or Dr Ron Stewart who introduced system changes born out of Los Angelas and Pittsburgh that led to a provincially integrated high-performance ground and air ambulance system (Geddes, Stewart and Baskett, 2017). As forever thankful to our physician mentors who advocated for changes within EMS systems and services we will be, updates to out-of-hospital patient care standards, system changes outside of the bricks and mortar of the hospital and challenging historical thinking was paramedic led. When we begin to unpack the history of paramedicine in Canada, we begin to take note of some significant landmarks. These notable landmarks are undoubtedly led by paramedic thinkers. Publications such as but not limited to the National Occupational Competency Profile (for paramedics), the National EMS Research Agenda (Jensen Socha, 2013), the Four Dimensions of Paramedic Practice in Canada: Defining and describing the profession (Bowles, vanBeek, Anderson, 2017) and the Principles and Enabling Factors Guiding Paramedicine in Canada (Tavares et. al., 2022). Arguably, the Emergency Medical Services Chiefs of Canada (known today as the Paramedic Chiefs of Canada, 2025), the Canadian Society of Ambulance Personnel (now known as the Paramedic Association of Canada) and the Canadian Organization of Paramedic Regulators all took the reins to lead in pushing judgement and decision making beyond that of their technician roots. Over the years across Canada, the term 'ambulance drivers' has all but been laid to rest.

Fast forward to today where paramedic scientists are making impacts to standards of care, paramedic educators are developing curriculum and teaching paramedics and other professional learners. There are paramedics using innovative technology such as AI, drones, and POCUS to deliver sophisticated care outside of and within a hospital. Across Canada you will still see variation from province to province on care provided to the community but rest assured licensed paramedics are now leading and mentoring other paramedics in the practice of paramedicine. If one were to compare stories from a paramedic in British Columbia to a paramedic on Prince Edward Island about the old days – there would be lots of variation in what is recalled and yet there are pieces that would resonate across the country. One thing that most would agree on, is that the evolution of paramedicine has happened at an alarming rate. Moving from a very technical job where attendants were told what to do, to that of a career that involves the ability to think critically, advocate for patients and make decisions based on risks, benefits and science. It is recognized and becoming widely accepted that paramedics are autonomous professionals that play a significant role in the journey of patients and families within and through the healthcare continuum. As healthcare and public safety demands change, so to do the demographics of patients and their disease and injury presentations. With the addition of more advanced providers and the need for more non-acute management, the standards to support an evolving patient demographic is also required. Today we continue to look to our paramedic leaders and thinkers to advocate for best practice, to deliver a high degree of patient and family centred care that is inclusive and impactful. This evolution has been astounding. From here, we will provide a glimpse into Canadian Paramedic advocacy including a brief look at the introduction of legislation to support the care delivered by paramedics.

Advocacy

In 1999, a national advocacy group of ambulance personnel began to explore and promote the idea of having certifications recognized from one province to the next within Canada. The idea of labour mobility led to the development of the Paramedic Association of Canada (PAC) shortly thereafter (PAC, 2025). In March 2000, PAC introduced the National Occupational Competency Profile (NOCP) for paramedics along with the professional titles of Primary Care Paramedic, Advanced Care Paramedic and Critical Care Paramedfic. The NOCP publication was one of the foundational documents that informed the evolution of paramedic practice today. The Paramedic Association of Canada continues to lobby the federal government in the promotion and advancement of the paramedic profession. Many provinces across Canada support the advocacy work of the Paramedic Association of Canada through provincial chapters.

In 2015, the Paramedic Association of Canada and Paramedic Chiefs of Canada agreed and anticipated a rapid evolution of paramedic practice across Canada. It was also surmised that preparation of paramedics for practice has not kept pace, and the depth and breadth of knowledge required to provide care to changing demographics of patients will soon extend beyond the scope of diploma education. The group committed to investigate and develop a plan for bachelor-degree education as an entry to practice requirement. In 2016, the Paramedic Association of Canada published the Paramedic Profile and Roles, Code of Ethics, Standards of Practice, and Education Guidance documents. This work was conducted as preparatory steps for a revised competency framework, wherein the paramedic community was invited to participate. This plan, known as 'Vision 2025' has progressed over the last decade, culminating in the development of the CSA Standard Z1660 National Competency Framework for Paramedics (NCFP) in 2024. This framework outlines the professional capabilities and opportunities for paramedics across five pathways within the profession: clinical practice, organizational leadership, research, education, and policy and strategy (Cameron and Batt, 2024).

The NCFP is aligned with the Paramedic Chief's of Canada's Principles to Guide the Future of Paramedicine. A suite of documents was further developed in 2024 aligned with the NCFP to reflect contemporary perspectives on the paramedic profession

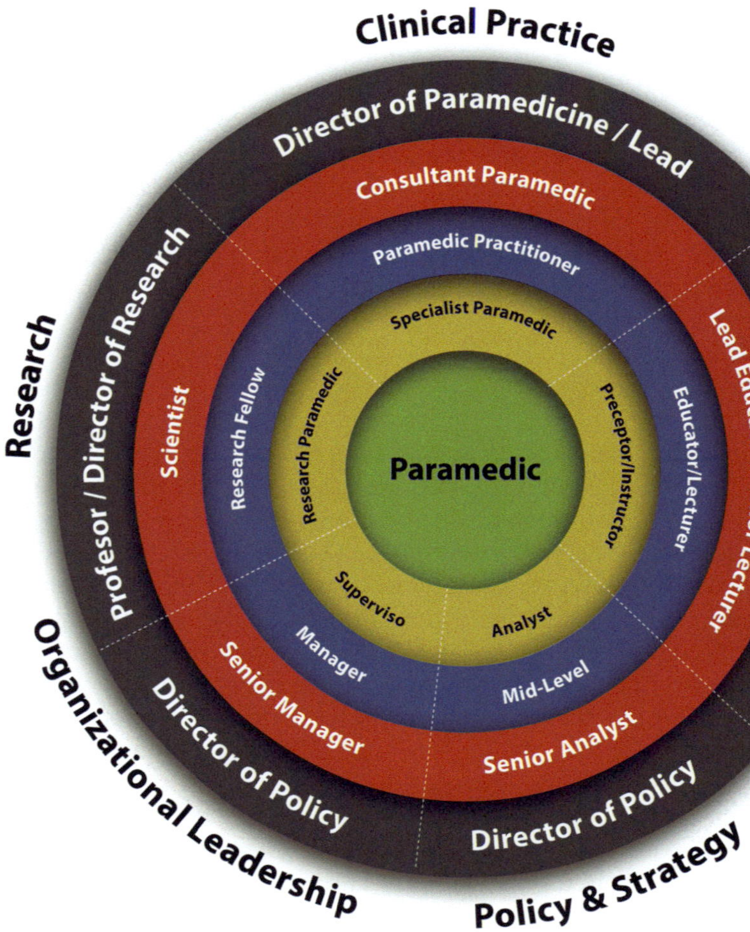

Figure 1.1 Career Framework for Paramedics
Source: Paramedic Association of Canada. Reproduced wtith permission.

in Canada. This includes the Career Framework for Paramedics. The NCFP, its supporting documents, and related specialist competency frameworks provide a solid foundation on which to develop bachelor-degree education, assessment, accreditation, and advanced practice roles in Canada.

Legislation and Regulation

In 2009, the Canadian Organization of Paramedic Regulators (COPR) formed. COPR serves two main purposes: to facilitate collective and collaborative action in the current and future interests of pan-Canadian paramedic regulation and to support the development of a common understanding of provincial and federal obligations that may impact regulator functions (COPR, 2025). COPR administers Entry to Practice Examinations for seven regulatory jurisdictions in Canada. In line with achieving professional regulation, the role of paramedic needed to develop into a truly professional one, in which members were held accountable for their actions and decisions. This evolution towards regulated practice that occurred in the early 2000s supported the notion that paramedics were considered as 'broadly autonomous', and implied significant responsibility to intervene with highly complex clinical scenarios, with little or no direct supervision by a physician. In 2021, COPR agreed to develop a harmonized and unified approach for pan-Canadian essential regulatory requirements: competencies and standards that will reflect and specifically focus on the needs of the public and patients for safe, effective care by paramedics.

In 2023, COPR released the Canadian Paramedic Competence Framework (CPCF). The framework describes current and actual practice, clarifies emergency medical responders' (EMRs) and paramedics' roles and responsibilities, and promotes consistency in measuring competence with a focus on patient safety and desired patient care outcomes. Each EMR and paramedic designation has its own framework, which collectively form the larger (CPCF) framework. Development in paramedicine comes with the responsibility to clearly describe what the public and patients can expect from a regulated paramedic to ensure safe, effective patient care. COPR's members, the provincial regulators for paramedicine, are committed to facilitating the framework's use to support consistent and uniform paramedic practice, regulation, and education in Canada.

Within the province of Nova Scotia (Canada). Paramedic practice is guided by legislation introduced and enacted on April 1, 2017 (College of Paramedic Nova Scotia, 2020). The Nova Scotia Paramedic Act and its associated Regulations protect the public and provide a blueprint for the practice of paramedicine within the province of Nova Scotia. Updates to this legislation and recent movement of the regulations within the Regulated Health Professions Act in Nova Scotia has significantly impacted the professionalism of paramedicine where paramedics are autonomous in their decision making and professional actions.

'Professionalism' can sometimes be a vague and somewhat nebulous term, often implied rather than bestowed, and with a sense that one can unconditionally adopt professionalism by dint of a qualification. While this may not be consistent with the emerging evidence, one could be forgiven for not fully appreciating what professionalism is. The Oxford English Dictionary has a comprehensive entry relating to the words 'professional' and 'professionalism' and includes reference to training, vocation, skill, knowledge, belonging (to a trade), conduct, income and standards (OED, 2013).

Being a member of a profession may not link to professionalism in all cases, but in healthcare, the values and behaviours which ensure that patients are treated effectively, safely and with dignity are vital to the point where professionalism exists as a feature alongside competent technical skill. Paramedics are, by definition, healthcare professionals and are registered and regulated accordingly. However, professionalism is achieved with a far more objective range of values, in many ways distinct from competency. For example, in the context of decision making, unprofessional behaviour may be seen when a patient, for whom admission to the Emergency Department is not indicated, is taken there by a paramedic who wants a cup of tea (which they know they can get there). In biomedical ethics, decisions about patients must demonstrate social justice, and the patient must never be the means to an end – they must only ever be the end in itself – to paraphrase Emanuel Kant (1724–1804). This means the value of the interaction with the patient must be derived from their needs rather than what the caregiver can gain (such as tea), and that the needs of the patient must be considered above other considerations. The patient should never be used as a means of achieving another goal – such as by leveraging the system to visit the place the paramedic wants to be (to get a cup of tea) rather than where the patient needs to be. Using the patient as a lever to visit the local hospital is unprofessional, and the decision making that leads to this is flawed.

We will explore throughout this book how the process of decision making is linked to other considerations, and professionalism is assumed throughout rather than being added as a constant reminder. It is important therefore to reflect on professionalism as a concept. This will promote optimal 'purity' in decision making, free from the extrinsic factors and stressors that may result in deviation from the focus essential to the patient–carer relationship. Basing practice on high professional standards makes decision making easier in many ways. It is an exercise that can be used to enhance professional fitness and therefore confidence and competence in practice.

The Evolving Role of Paramedics and Changing Practice Settings

The paramedic role is evolving rapidly with greater opportunity to practice across a range of settings spanning the career framework, and with far more mobility than previously experienced by paramedics. Prior to the start of the new millennium, roles for paramedics rarely extended beyond employment in an ambulance service, either in clinical roles or as managers or trainers. Indeed, in many parts of the country until even relatively recent times, paramedics were in a minority of the ambulance service's clinical workforce, but also there were limited, if any, opportunities for clinical development beyond this role.

The changing expectations, operational roles and scope of practice in paramedicine have a direct impact on both educational content and educational practice. Paramedic educators seeking to prepare practitioners for these roles face an intriguing set of challenges. Some of these new roles bring paramedics' existing scope of practice to new environments. Other roles are opportunities for paramedics with expanded scopes of practice to provide alternative forms of care within their existing context of practice. Changes in patient disposition and treatment options radically change the types of decisions paramedics will make, and the educational foundation needed to function effectively. (Bowles et al, 2017) Higher education in Canadian paramedicine is work on the horizon and greatly needed to support the type of decisions that will be expected of professional paramedics currently and in the future.

Prior to the protected titles of paramedics, decision making often extended only as far as applying basic treatments and deciding which hospital was closest. However, paramedic practice has continued to develop in the twenty-first century, highlighting the need for a more consistent professional career framework, underpinned by better education and training for those joining the profession. Principles to Guide the Future of Paramedicine in Canada (2022) makes reference to the need to advance the depth and breadth of knowledge in the system from entry to practice to leadership, as a means to achieve many future desired states. Advancing knowledge, skills, competencies, and expertise through higher education across domains such as clinical care, social sciences, humanities, leadership, economics, quality, research, technologies, and logistics, were believed to enable bridges to the future goals of paramedicine. At the time of printing for this edition, a province within Canada is undertaking a project to implement the work associated with the NCFP and encouraging education institutions to ensure education and curriculum is aligned with the proposed career framework. Other Canadian provinces are making strides to implement higher education within paramedicine beyond the historical diploma offerings.

The fact that paramedics are no longer synonymous only with ambulances or ambulance services is good news for patients and the profession. The support given to the paramedic professional, such as in the *Urgent and Emergency Care Review* produced by Professor Sir Bruce Keogh, Medical Director for NHS England between 2013 and 2018, has given paramedics roles in a much wider range of practice settings (NHS England, 2013). While there remains a predominance for paramedics to commence their careers within the ambulance service, paramedics can work in emergency departments, industrial settings, correctional settings, aeromedical services, clinics and military healthcare. The career opportunities for those entering the profession are rich and diverse, and the breadth of settings often include much more inter-professional and multi-professional working, with teams formed from other allied health professionals, nurses and doctors, as well as mental health professionals, social care professionals and other agencies' staff. Paramedics do not just work alongside the police and fire brigade anymore, and are positioned firmly as health professionals.

In order to be trusted as a healthcare professional, it is vital for paramedics to be seen as decision makers so as to represent themselves consistently according to their core professional identity. The breadth of opportunities that exist can help ensure patients have the best access to high quality care from a range of skilled healthcare professionals, each with their own unique skills and abilities, coming together to define the nature of multi-professionalism. Conversely, the risk of making healthcare professions generic may dilute the unique core skills of paramedics, as well as those of the other health professions. All these professions potentially run the risk of being viewed as interchangeable because of the apparent similarity of intent when providing care. In turn, this may damage the patient/carer relationship. Arguably, the uniqueness of a paramedic lies in being an immediate care clinician, who has a combination of emergency and generalist knowledge and provides a calm and collected approach to any situation – scheduled or unscheduled – towards reaching a care resolution with the patient. These attributes are desirable for decision makers, particularly when under pressure.

It is worth noting that, internationally, paramedic practice is evolving. Australian paramedic practice now also has (or is working towards) a formal regulatory body; the same is true in New Zealand. Paramedic science research is performed in other areas of the world too, such as the Americas (Martin & O'Meara, 2019; Martínez et al., 2018; Becker et al., 2017), Africa (Gage et al., 2020; Abwalaba & Onyango, 2019; Oboro et al., 2015) and Asia (Nik Muhamad, 2020; Harari et al., 2019), demonstrating how valuable paramedics can be to any healthcare system. While the purpose of this edition of the book is to predominantly focus on Canadian practice, it is hoped that other paramedics will observe similarities (and differences) of decision making that can be extrapolated to their realm of practice.

Patient Demography and Epidemiology

Paramedics are seeing patients in an increasingly wide range of practice settings in Canada, such as ambulance services, industrial clinics, in the community and within emergency departments.

Paramedics who practice in any sector of the healthcare continuum that involve the management of patients with long-term conditions, regardless of them being seen for ongoing care or for an acute presentation, should be aware of the importance of appreciating any potential knowledge gap in the understanding of the impact of underlying health conditions (for example, managing a patient with type 1 diabetes who develops an infection).

Underpinning all of these considerations, paramedics are most commonly decision makers in the acute phase of care, and often face a multitude of clinical presentations that range from self-resolving minor illness, to exacerbation of chronic disease, to multi-morbid deterioration. Individuals, as patients in that moment, are anticipating an appropriate decision, no matter how complex.

Paramedic education covers a wide range of clinical scenarios and builds confidence in the management of life-threatening or other serious conditions. However, there are conditions, circumstances and presentations that commonly cause anxiety among paramedics when it comes to decision making; for instance, areas such as paediatrics, obstetric care, mental health and end of life care are becoming hot topics for employers' on-going training and support, as well as paramedics' self-directed CPD.

For paramedics, contact with patients often occurs at times of crisis and therefore these encounters are complex. Decision making in relation to the **co-morbid** patient suffering an acute-on-chronic presentation may also involve considerations relating to advanced decisions and end of life care. Later chapters look at the dilemmas and conundrums faced in practice, and discuss scenarios relating to patients with long-term healthcare needs.

Activity – Understanding Acuity and Complexity

The profile of patients that paramedics come across in their role has changed in line with both the epidemiology and indices of deprivation in our communities and the breadth of places where paramedics see their patients. As already discussed, previously the types of patients that paramedics encountered were high acuity, but were perhaps lower in complexity (diseases and treatment options).

When considering acuity in the context of decision-making, it is helpful to consider the wider picture that comprises the overall impression of acuity. Using the following three grids you can mentally map the patient's acuity and complexity objectively, and use this information to guide your management and treatment plan.

Grid 1: Basic Acuity of the Disease Presentation (Onset vs Severity)

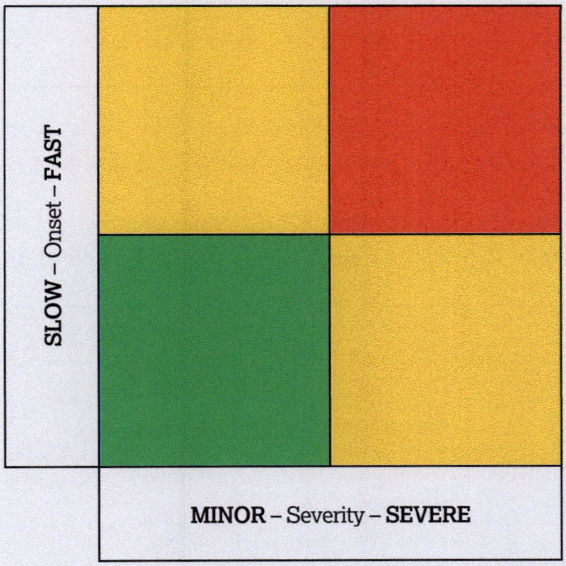

Once you have an awareness of the level of acuity, the complexity can be considered. Complexity in engineering terms is commonly assessed by considering the number of moving parts. For example, a bicycle may be considered relatively simple when compared to a Formula 1 car or a helicopter. In a healthcare context, complexity includes factors such as the number of diseases present and other underlying patient factors, such as age, social history, allergies and frailty.

Grid 2: Assessment of Complexity (Existing Diseases vs Patient Factors)

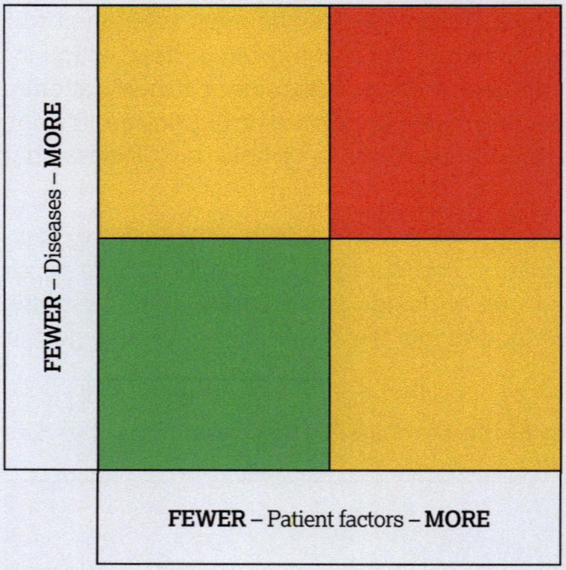

Placing your patient in an acuity/complexity grid can assist with your decision making when considering your limitations or the limitations of the environment or system you are in.

Grid 3: Assessment of Acuity vs Complexity (Based on Grid 1 and Grid 2)

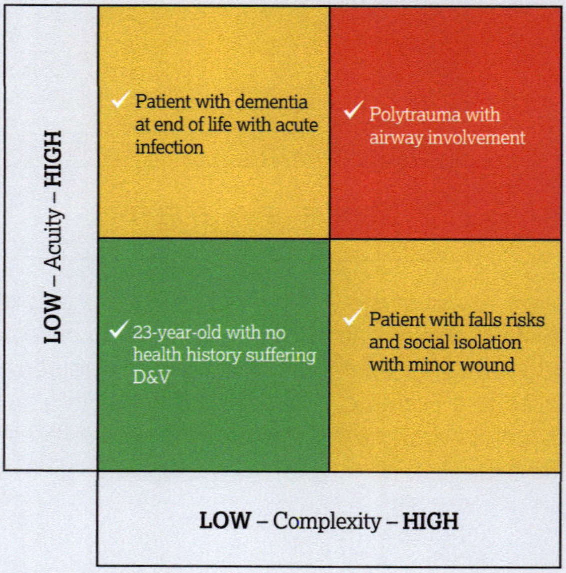

Grid 3 has some example conditions in each cell. Where would you put the following scenarios?

- 24-year-old male with a twisted ankle.
- 92-year-old female with type 1 diabetes and heart failure who has a 3-day history of dysuria.
- 33-year-old male involved in a high-speed road traffic collision. Head, chest and pelvic injuries. Reduced level of consciousness. Not ventilating adequately.

Why not revisit this exercise once you have finished the book to see if you would think differently.

People with long term conditions consistently say:

- They want to be involved in decisions about their care – they want to be listened to.
- They want access to information to help them make those decisions.
- They want support to understand their condition and confidence to manage – support to self-care.
- They want joined up, seamless services.
- They want proactive care.
- They do not want to be in hospital unless it is absolutely necessary and then only as part of a planned approach.
- They want to be treated as a whole person.

(DH, 2012: 3)

Patients with long-term healthcare problems are a growing cohort and are usually complex. Improving the approach to decision making for this group of patients is vital for paramedics if they are to contribute effectively to the health of the nation and to support healthcare policy in action – most importantly ensuring that patients' voices are heard, and their wishes met. Long-term disease prevalence and multi-morbidity cannot, however, be seen in isolation; there are two more important aspects to care – ageing and deprivation – which impact on decision making and often exist alongside long-term healthcare problems as a triad.

Ageing in itself is not a disease, but the anatomical, physiological and psychological changes experienced in ageing are important to underlying health. Older patients are more prone to illness, often associated with age and the risk of, or presence of, frailty. This results in patients living independently or in supported living in the community, doing so with increased risks to their health, secondary to their age or other factors. For instance, an older patient with diminished bone density and **polypharmacy** is at far higher risk of falling and suffering a fracture. Patients who have already suffered a fracture over the age of 65 are far more likely to suffer another 'fragility fracture' as a result of subsequent falls. Patients in this group are often also on novel oral anticoagulants (NOACs), which increase the risk of bleeding, both externally and internally. The decision making for this group of patients, therefore, is increasingly complex – considering carefully the risk–benefit balance of promoting independent living versus admission to hospital in the face of increased risk of an injurious fall. This can only be done in the presence of good decision making that ensures the patient is paramount and their wishes are considered in the context of the information they need to make an informed decision about their own healthcare.

Decision making has many cues and places from which better-formed ideas can be tested. Consideration must be given to all the factors that assist with making a better decision. Working in certain areas or working with certain defined groups (such as by age or deprivation), consideration can be given to increasing the context of care in these settings, and while this is not the main influence in making a decision, it helps with the richness of the analysis and therefore the quality of the result for the patient.

Conclusion

Paramedic practice has an increasingly strong identity and a unique selling point as a dependable clinical problem solver. The evolution of paramedicine and paramedic practice is happening at an alarming rate. Paramedics are working across healthcare at an increasing scale in settings such as the ambulance sector and the myriad other multi-professional practice settings, emergency departments, military, offshore, in the community and within critical care transport. Decision making must be one of the cornerstones of professional practice as it underpins and promotes safety during clinical encounters – regardless of the practice setting. The early understanding of ambulance work across this nation was largely predicated on the concept of rapid assessment and early transport to a hospital for treatment. As we sunset legacy documents, titles and terminology, and we begin to produce an evidence informed body of knowledge, how paramedics practice has evolved tremendously. One may suggest there is an opportunity to include decision making as a part of curriculum within higher paramedic education programs going forward to support this evolution with paramedicine. Without objective decision making, any imbalance between confidence and competence can be dangerous; therefore, professional responsibility and autonomy should be considered carefully in the context of self-awareness and the risks associated with biased thinking.

Patient-centred care means that all healthcare professionals need to strive to make the safest and most appropriate decisions about each individual patient's care, and these decisions must be reached on the basis that the patient is paramount. As professional practice has developed and become more complex, healthcare professionals must become better at decision making in order to create the best outcome for patients.

Reflective Exercises

1. Consider your own role in clinical practice and reflect on your own professional development, taking into account the ageing population and the increasingly complex patients for whom paramedics provide care.
2. What do professional and regulatory standards mean to you? Consider the key pan-Canadian Essential Regulatory Requirement documents published by the Canadian Organization of Paramedic Regulators at this stage of your development in relation to making decisions. (You may want to repeat this reflective exercise after reading Chapter 6.)
3. What does it mean to be an Allied Healthcare Professional? In relation to decision making, what similarities and differences are there between professions?

Chapter 2

Professional and Ethical Issues

Si Robinson and Andy Collen

Chapter Objectives

This chapter will cover:

- Professional regulation and standards
- Professional identity
- Decision making through the lens of bioethics
- Patient-centred care
- Confidentiality – the crossroads between professionalism and bioethics
- Competence and confidence in practice
- Professional insight.

Introduction

In order to deliver care and decisions for, and with, your patients and other healthcare professionals, it is important to fully understand the constellation of other factors and considerations which guide and regulate professional practice. Many of the aspects discussed in this chapter are indirectly related to decision-making theory, providing fundamental concepts to consider and reflect upon as intrinsic aspects of day-to-day clinical practice as a paramedic. These foundations ensure that the care you provide, including every decision, is directly or indirectly in line with published standards, ethical considerations, laws and legislation, evidence-based guidance, and patient-focused principles. Personal integrity plays a significant role in professional practice; displaying insight into your practice helps to weave together your knowledge, skills and competencies into a **holistic acumen** upon which good decisions can be built.

Professional clinical practice involves a significant amount of personal sacrifice, study, long hours, bearing witness to traumatic and stressful events and, most importantly, being registered with a regulating body. This is balanced against the privilege of being invited into patients' lives at their time of need, seeking to find an initial resolution that will better their situation in some way, such as administering life-saving interventions, making them comfortable at the end of their life, or simply listening to their concerns and providing reassurance.

Something that is almost unique to paramedic practice is serving as one of the first clinicians a patient will see, which provides a vital window of opportunity to ensure that what happens next – broadly, to signpost, refer on or offer advice are the correct courses of action. This notion is a form of **gatekeeping**, where a paramedic has the tough decision of ensuring that the following action will be of benefit to the patient while not at the cost of using limited resources. However, the risk of harm and error behind this decision needs to remain minimal, yet is incredibly difficult to measure, where the consequence of making a poor decision can quite literally be life or death, and this can be overwhelming for paramedics.

For instance, it is well documented that paramedics frequently make the decision to convey a patient to hospital, as it is often considered the safest (and least risky) course of action (Miles et al., 2019; O'Hara et al., 2015). While most decisions to admit are correct, the decision must be in the patient's best interest and be clinically appropriate; hospital colleagues are already under pressure, there is risk of exposing a patient to hospital-acquired infection or iatrogenic harm, and further tests may be conducted that are unnecessary. Telling a patient that hospital admission is not appropriate may result in conflict, disempowerment, moral distress and reduced trust and access with other healthcare services. In older patients or frail patients, hospital admission can lead to deconditioning and impact on recovery and rehabilitation, and may even lead to worsening health (BGS, 2017). A patient should not attend hospital if they do not need to; nor should you, as a paramedic, be expected to convey a patient merely because they demand it.

These potential outcomes both exemplify poor forms of gatekeeping, where much of the art of being a good clinician (and decision maker) is about striking the balance between delivering care that acts in the patient's best interests with professional integrity, while maintaining patient expectation and limiting risk or error. These are key themes that are uncovered throughout this chapter (and book).

To be an effective clinician, it is vital to promote confidence in your practice. There are plenty of opportunities to create anxiety in oneself as a clinician – particularly associated with making complex decisions, and that often insidious threat (perceived or actual) of consequences when things go wrong. We will explore some of these factors in the context of decision making and reflecting how to further understand and minimize risk, particularly relating to professional considerations. It is extremely rare for errors to be made intentionally – no one comes to work to do a bad job. Where problems arise, judgements are made more commonly in the context of reasonable actions and opportunities to learn. Being prepared, competent, and able to make defensible decisions – rather than practising defensively – is a way of ensuring your clinical practice is safe and rewarding.

There are a range of issues involving decision making, and these include concepts such as patient-centred care, confidentiality, impartiality, biomedical ethics and reflection. This chapter will link these areas of learning, and the concepts presented, in the context of these considerations. This chapter is intended to add colour to your emerging and developing decision-making acumen, ensuring that one avoids becoming a 'decision-making robot', and retains the safe holistic approach to care that our patients deserve, with an awareness of the wider professional factors that are not always at the forefront of our minds.

Professional Regulation and Standards

As highlighted in the introductory chapter, the Canadian Organization of Paramedic Regulators have published the Regulatory Practice Standards (the 'Standards'). These standards are available to guide paramedics and EMRs, provincial regulatory organizations, and paramedicine educators by describing the outcomes of the minimal performance standards expected of paramedics and EMRs in Canada, regardless of their designation, job description, or practice setting. For example, a paramedic educator modelling treatment while teaching a learner is expected to meet the requirements set out in the standards. The Standards serve to promote the consistency of entry to practice requirements across Canada and to support labour mobility. Although not all provinces within Canada have adopted these Standards, many have used the COPR Standards to support or inform legislation and public expectation pertaining to paramedic practice (COPR, 2025).

Activity

As a quick test, can you name the ten regulatory practice standards published by COPR? Do you know where to find them if you can't? (See appendix for answer.)

The purpose of all healthcare professional regulators, such as the Nova Scotia Regulator of Paramedicine (NSRoP, 2025), is to protect the public, not to serve its registrants. The NSRoP along with the other regulators regulators that are included within the Regulated Health Professions Act (RHP Act, 2024) are given oversight and scrutiny by the Nova Scotia Government, and all work to ensure that registrants uphold and follow the standards stated by each regulator.

All regulators publish their register. This allows members of the public to check if their healthcare professional is registered and/or subject to any conditions or sanctions. Importantly, employers can check whether their staff are registered, and work with regulators in cases involving their own staff members. Regulation should not be confused with membership of a professional body or a trade union, and the financial element of registration is an inevitable aspect of professional practice, as these registration forms need to be maintained. The other key role of the professional regulator is to ensure that the protected titles associated with registered professions are not misused. This means that the regulator has the power to bring prosecutions against those who use protected titles without being registered. This is a very important aspect of registration and links closely to professional identity, which in turn provides further assurance to the public that the healthcare professionals providing their care are registered, authentic and practising to minimum standards.

Scope of Practice: Individual Skills, Specialty or Organizational Policy?

A fundamental term synonymous with regulation is scope of practice. Among the regulations and standards, this term is perhaps the most important yet most vague. Its importance cannot be overstated, as practising beyond one's scope places the public in danger. However, scope can be difficult to define as paramedics practise at differing levels (primary care, advanced care and critical care) and in different settings (primary care, pre-hospital, hospital), and develop additional skills and specialist knowledge (for example, wound closure, ultrasound, casting, palliative care, paediatrics, critical care). Below are some key examples.

Example 1: Intubation

Endotracheal intubation (ETI) and airway management remains a core component within paramedic scope of practice. Yet, with growing evidence (Edwards, 2017), ETI in practice is now shifting towards paramedics in roles where it is more frequently implemented: the critical care specialty and setting. This has resulted in some organizations limiting paramedics at non-advanced levels from performing ETI, in favour of supraglottic airway devices, thus restricting individual scope of practice and competence maintenance. While some individuals irrespective of level may feel that they are perfectly competent to perform ETI based on the situation, this example demonstrates how professional specialism and organizational policy, based on evidential guidance, serves to add layers that protect the public from harm.

Example 2: Specialist Interest in a Particular Field

Perhaps the hardest scope to regulate, is where an individual develops specialist knowledge within a specific field or subset, for example in procedural sedation and analgesia (PSA) in the emergency department, gaining increased understanding and confidence of the sedation continuum, sedation risk factors and pharmacology. With the enhanced knowledge the individual may be able to base decisions that are perceptively risky within the organization and to other non-specialized paramedics, yet entirely justified and evidentially best practice. The regulations and licensure encourages continued professional development, placing responsibility with the individual to evidence learning and competence. This example relates back to autonomy, where specialist interests ought to be supported, as it is one of the fundamental elements that motivates individuals, establishes organizational commitment and drives the profession forward (Hobbs et al., 2021; Hodge et al., 2018; Bartlett, 2001). However, it is important to note that not all paramedics feel this way, with a preference to be externally guided by an organization in career development as opposed to intrinsic motivation (Hobbs et al., 2021).

Scope of practice can therefore be argued as limitless but contextually bounded (see Figure 2.1). The above-mentioned paramedic with PSA specialism for instance, may have the knowledge and skill to perform a sedation; at the individual and professional level, this demonstrates fantastic capacity to evolve practice (applied to pre-hospital cardiac arrest for instance – Reed et al., 2017), yet must be suitably negotiated and applied within their role within the organization. Despite evidence for paramedic-led decision-making are anesthetizing patients, performing PSA in an out-of-hospital space would be unsafe practice if not sanctioned by an organization. As such, stepping beyond the bounded context, in this case organizational but possibly also individual competence or professional role, ought to lead to a fitness to practise review by the regulatory body in the interest of safe patient care.

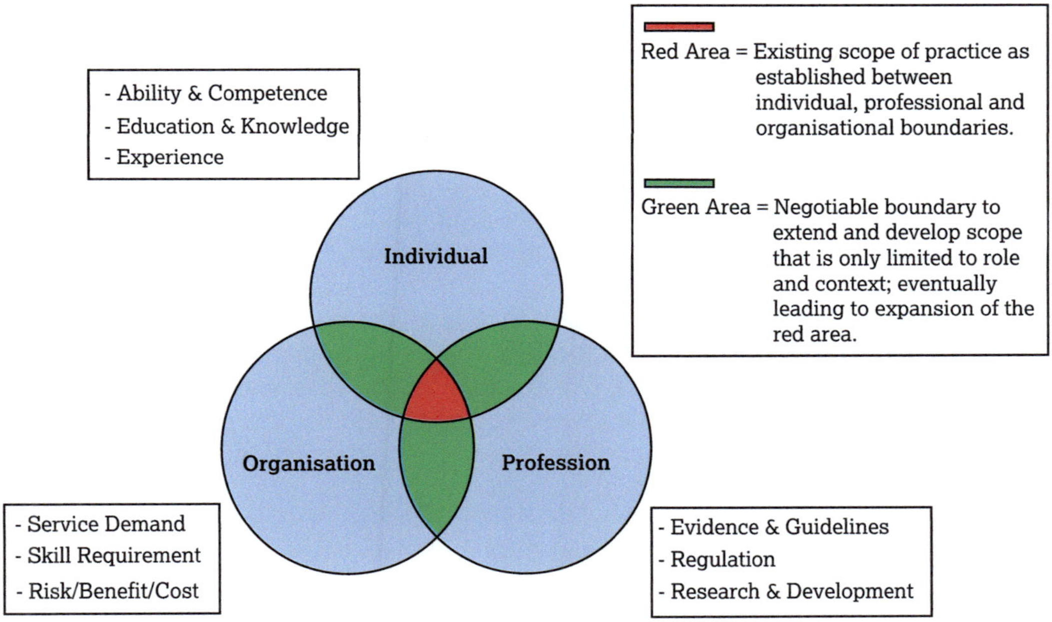

Figure 2.1 Scope of practice within context.
Source: Si Robinson

Fitness to Practise and Sanctions

Within the regulated health profession fitness to practise (FTP) concerns are usually brought forward to the regulatory body. Concerns may solely relate to a breach of scope of practice; they may also be due to health concerns, misconduct (such as dishonesty, deliberate harm or negligence) or a lack of competency (a failure to be able to practise to an acceptable standard). In other words, the HCPTS do not seek to apply a punishment considering acts or omissions, but in the rare instance where the issue is serious enough to warrant a sanction, suspension or condition to be applied to a paramedic license. This clearly by its nature may end up being punitive.

An FTP referral may occur from a service user, another professional or member of the organization, or as a self-referral.

It is important to remember that the application of sanctions is primarily to ensure the public are assured that the profession is fit to practise, and also that the reputation of the profession is upheld.

We will cover being confident in practice later in this chapter; however, in the context of decision-making, the statistics that relate to paramedic complaints and concerns made to the regulator should be reflected upon as the reality of professional practice. Regulation means that you should not approach your professional role with fear of the regulator, instead the published standards should be used to guide you alongside your own values, morals and standards. It is important to remember that paramedics often practise in extremely hostile practice environments, and therefore any lapses of judgement may be exacerbated by situational or other **human factors** (such as poorly designed work system, stress, fatigue or work intensity).

Professional Identity

Professional identity is defined by Ashforth, Harrison and Corley as the 'essential human desire to expand the self-concept to include connections with others and to feel a sense of belonging with a larger group' (Ashforth et al., 2008). In essence, newcomers to paramedic practice are socialized into the profession role, developing a distinguished identity that shares attributes, values, motives and experiences (Gallagher et al., 2016; Ibarra, 1999). These characteristics are thought to distinguish the paramedic profession from being perceived as merely an occupation, as well as providing an identity separate from other healthcare professions, such as medicine or nursing.

Historically, sociologists such as Goode (1960) and Barber (1963) adopted a functionalist approach in identifying professional traits, where the profession in question fulfils a vital role necessary to the functioning of society. Traits such as 'prolonged specialist training in a body of abstract knowledge' (Goode, 1960, p. 903), 'a concern for interests in the community' (Barber, 1963, p. 672), 'a code of ethics' (Barber, 1963, p. 672), and 'members more strongly identify with their profession than members of other occupations' (Goode, 1960, p. 903) have been suggested as core elements that define a profession. However, the functionalist construct ignores issues such as the power dynamics between competing professions, and assumes (and justifies) a status quo (such as doctors are the archetypical healthcare profession). To remedy these issues, Freidson (2001), perhaps one of the most important contributors to the notion of socialized professionalism, particularly to healthcare, identified key characteristics that define a professional identity separate from other or competing professions. Broadly, these are:

1. A specialist degree of knowledge and skills involved in professional work that non-professionals are unable to evaluate.

2. That professionals are autonomous and can be trusted to work unsupervised.
3. The profession can regulate themselves.

For paramedics, it is easy to see that operating in a pre-hospital ambulance setting fits Freidson's theory. Indeed, Ruth Townsend in her thesis (2017) used this as a platform to contribute towards regulation for Australian paramedics, since it makes for a powerful argument justifying paramedics as a professional entity. Although not emphasized in Chapter 1, paramedic education is followed by an application of learning in a preceptorship environment. Success in preceptorship is required before writing an entry to practice examination before autonomy is attained. Paramedic regulations (and paramedics therein) regulates the profession, and the Paramedic Association of Canada guides it. There are, however, issues that arguably diminish the paramedic discipline as a profession.

Historically, much of the specialist knowledge relating to paramedic practice was guided and underwritten by the medical profession. This has resolved over the last decade or more in light of the growing body of evidence that pre-hospital care differs significantly from an in-hospital setting, as well as the highly complementary relationship between the paramedic profession and medicine (see Ebben et al., 2020; Höglund et al., 2020; Grunwald et al., 2020; van Dongen et al., 2019; Lockey et al., 2015 as examples, although there are many more), and by this, the emphasis may be on stabilization and rapid conveyance as opposed to the use of diagnostic equipment to secure a diagnosis. To a degree, this dynamic is changing with the growing body of evidence that paramedics themselves are establishing through science and evidence.

Paramedics are becoming synonymous with urgent and emergency care in their diverse practice settings and also remain the predominant expert profession in the ambulance setting. There are ongoing research studies to understand the role and influence of medicine in prehospital care and how this can be used to further strengthen multi-professional practice to the benefit of patients.[1]

An additional issue is that paramedics have the option to study and develop beyond the ambulance into areas such as emergency departments, tactical teams, rapid response teams and community clinics. These settings require paramedics to work within multidisciplinary teams, challenging the concept and status quo as to what differentiates a paramedic from a nurse, a doctor or a physician assistant. This is not unique to paramedic practice and affects all professions that are related in some way to healthcare. Due in part to the increasing service demand, and in turn

[1] There is a strong counter-argument that maintaining a diverse workforce in any care setting breaks down hierarchical and professional boundaries, fostering collaboration from each respective discipline that drives innovation and new models of care. This is discussed later on in this chapter. Perhaps the point here is less on professional dominance and more on the significant relationship a paramedic has within the pre-hospital domain, representing the bulk of the registered clinical workforce in the UK.

lack of clinicians (traditionally the shortfall in medical staffing) to meet these needs, the opportunity for alternative professions to adapt and evolve arises, with some inevitable crossover.

For instance, paramedics as well as nurses have been recognized as versatile professions that can meet this shortfall, particularly in frontline settings such as primary, urgent, community and emergency care. In the case of emergency medicine, both professions can specialize as advanced clinical practitioners remaining regulated under their respective bodies yet sharing exactly the same scope of practice. This demonstrates that the paramedic profession has the attributes, expertise and capability in filling the gaps in which the medical profession struggles to deliver, offering paramedics new scope and specialist interests they are not often exposed to in the ambulance setting. Consequently, professional boundaries are blurred, confronting these core characteristics and, therefore, the identity of a paramedic.

Before addressing the issues that challenge professionalism and exploring how and indeed if the characteristics of a paramedic remain despite a change in role and setting, let us explore in further detail the notion of autonomy and regulation.

Autonomy

Healthcare practice has in some ways developed a currency around the term 'autonomy'. Simply meaning to 'self-govern', the value in both autonomous individuals and a profession as a whole is the ability to rely on tasks to be completed without the need for supervision. In healthcare, this relinquishes the senior clinician (a base hospital physician or medical oversight physician, for instance) from having to micro-manage every element of the patient journey. This approach enables layers of clinicians to make decisions that in turn reduce the demand of senior input while retaining a timely, safe and cost-effective method of care delivery.

As previously discussed, paramedics primarily act as a form of gatekeeper, with the capability to triage an individual based on clinical assessment and to manage accordingly. This concept of filtering may be of use here in Canada to minimize excessive input from primary and emergency care clinicians, while increasing the autonomy of paramedics.

Paramedics are expected to be autonomous, to further develop with more autonomy in advanced practice, and respect the autonomy of service users. The latter point will be discussed later under ethics; the former highlights how paramedic practice can be a confusing environment to make self-governing decisions. In a critical care situation for instance, it is preferable to work as a team and share decisions, yet in a low acuity scenario it could be perfectly acceptable to manage as a lone worker. Moreover, since the advent of checklists and scoring systems such as NEWS2, which can reinforce decisions and improve patient safety (Scott et al., 2020; Martín-Rodríguez et al., 2019), little is known of whether such tools impede autonomy or the ability to think 'outside the box' in atypical situations. A prime example would be applying a NEWS2 score to an individual approaching the end of life, where vital signs are typically deranged. Therefore, where autonomy intersects with teamwork, guidelines, and individual ability, complexity is introduced or increased. Perhaps therefore it is better to focus on the use of autonomy in its most positive light: freedom to think and freedom to act but within clear boundaries, which serve to promote patient safety and optimal outcomes.

Case Example

There has been a growing body of evidence that the risk of applying a cervical spine collar in suspected spinal injury outweighs any benefit (Hawkridge et al., 2020; Hodgett and Ward, 2020). Nonetheless, guidelines have become increasingly fragmented as evidence emerges regarding the application of collars in suspected spinal injury subject to the Canadian C-Spine Rule (a decision aide) and sensitivity towards pre-existing spinal pathology (National Institute of Health and Care Excellence, 2024). The decision to apply one therefore requires consideration. For example, based on assessment, a paramedic may decide that a less invasive or more conservative approach would yield greater benefit; this is particularly the case for head injuries and children where a semi-rigid collar is associated with other problems. Therefore, the paramedic has operated autonomously based on knowledge of both cervical spine pathology and cervical collars, guidelines and decision-aides, patient safety and interests to deliver effective care despite partially deviating from guidelines (note that in the case of children, manual stabilization is advised). Suppose, however, that this decision was challenged by a colleague on scene or at the hospital. The ability to justify the decision, engage in a discussion, or even change or trial an alternative suggestion is the essence of autonomy, and the example of cervical collars illustrates how important and apparent such a concept is in paramedic practice at an individual and team level.

So, in accordance with Freidson's theory, paramedics must be autonomous, but also recognize when to balance this against teamwork, guidelines and shared decisions. What about the development and progression of autonomy, such as following a course or framework extending knowledge and scope of practice?

The concept of increasing autonomy has several issues including the context of specialist knowledge acquisition, and the application thereof, which has implications to both the patient and the profession. Studying a Master's in critical care would certainly improve knowledge within that field, but not, say, the management of long-term conditions. Similarly, a critical care paramedic would not have any more authority in managing a suspected urinary tract infection than a regular paramedic, yet an urgent care specialist/paramedic practitioner would.

As an example, the Royal College of Paramedics, alongside NHS England Workforce Training and Education (as well as equivalent organizations in the devolved nations), has devised frameworks that enable paramedics in the UK to evidence their scope of clinical practice. The newly qualified paramedic portfolio is arguably the beginning of this journey, encouraging paramedics to build evidence and examples of autonomous decision making and robust clinical practice. Following this, paramedics have an opportunity to discover their particular interests, begin to build upon them with additional courses and training, and pursue alternative roles within or beyond the ambulance service setting. This is a key component of continued professional development that is regulated and will be discussed shortly. Although not mandatory, progressing to specialist and advanced practice is determined by an extensive portfolio that covers the 'four pillars' of advanced practice devised by Health Education England (2017) (now NHSE): clinical practice, research, leadership and management, and education. Evidencing autonomy falls under clinical practice, which bears relevance to the specific advanced practice setting. Primarily for paramedics, this is within primary care, urgent and emergency care, pre-hospital and critical care.

To enable clarity of paramedic status, level of autonomy and specialty both to other professionals and to patients, a simple solution is for roles including specialist and advanced ones to be appropriately titled (which is often the case): primary care paramedic, advanced care paramedic, critical care paramedic, community care paramedic and so on. The alternative for advanced roles, is to amalgamate advanced practice to a single titular role, such as the aforementioned 'advanced clinical practitioner', irrespective of original healthcare background. As previously discussed, this blurs role boundaries and may create a professional identity crisis. Fortunately, where advanced clinical practitioners form a breadth of professions working together, core role features do remain and serve only to further enhance the quality of the care provided.

Although multi-professional roles with a common postgraduate education base have become embedded within the healthcare system, it is important to celebrate and promote the uniqueness each profession has to offer. This ensures professional identity and prevents patients being confused about who is providing their care.

Further, as in medicine or nursing, the more one leans towards a specific specialty, the harder it is to transfer across to another without taking some form of a career step backwards or additional learning. Likewise, with the increasing autonomy of an advanced practitioner, multiple settings could potentially benefit from the extended scope. The model of rotational paramedic practice, working in a variety of settings, such as primary care, urgent care, the ambulance and telehealth, demonstrates promise that a multitude of settings would benefit from the enhanced autonomy specialist and advanced paramedics can provide (Creton et al., 2020; Turner and Williams, 2018).

Autonomy is important for healthcare professionals to evidence and plays an important role in both the development of the paramedic profession within the growing plurality of professions that exist within a multitude of settings and the day-to-day decisions therein. Professional autonomy is not to be misconstrued as the Kantian concept of 'freedom from external control or influence', which relates to ethical autonomy; such a concept does not exist in professional healthcare, as external influences, such as governments, patient advocacy groups, clinical commissioning groups and economics, are all contributory factors that shape the healthcare landscape to which paramedic practice resides (see Light, 2010, for a further discussion).[2] Thus, autonomy should not be perceived as limited within a hierarchy, where paramedics operate somewhere among doctors, nurses and healthcare assistants, limited in scope and destined to handover or delegate decisions. Instead, autonomy is a means to transform as an individual decision maker that represents the paramedic profession. One that garners trust, is involved and engaged and able to integrate and negotiate care decisions among patients and other healthcare professionals.

Summarizing the Notion of Professional Identity

It was highlighted earlier that paramedics are no longer synonymous with pre-hospital care, and that beyond the ambulance and with advancing practice, professional boundaries become increasingly blurred. Freidson (2001) argued that a profession must be autonomous, self-regulating and attain a high degree of specialist knowledge for it to establish itself within society.

For paramedics, this is no longer confined to the pre-hospital setting; the specialist knowledge attained is to be a first point-of-contact healthcare professional, one that is incredibly versatile. Very few healthcare professionals have the ability to deliver a baby, perform resuscitation, manage an acute exacerbation of a chronic condition, reassure a lonely elderly person, perform a mental health assessment and offer advice for a minor illness such as rhinosinusitis. It is these elements that attract additional sectors, such as primary care or rapid response teams, to employ paramedics.

So, the future of paramedic practice is to be identified as an expert first-contact clinician. Perhaps the first healthcare professional an individual consults with, or within a team of other healthcare professionals,[3] versatile in knowledge with limitless avenues to explore specialist interests provided they meet regulatory standards. Certainly, the term 'first contact' is anticipated to be increasingly used among paramedics in healthcare – NHSE announced the First Contact Practitioner Paramedic Framework (Health Education England, 2021) for developing paramedics in primary care, and this term could expand to additional settings, such as urgent

---

[2] Although beyond the scope of this book, this interplay can be seen globally by exploring the similarities and differences of paramedic roles and practice in different countries and continents.

[3] Indeed, the term paramedic literally means 'beside medicine', which can be expanded to 'beside all healthcare professionals'. Rather than be perceived as an adjunct to medicine (this lens will always render paramedic practice as inferior to medicine, and arguably anybody that adheres to this model will either feel restricted or wonder whether they should have studied medicine, a completely different profession), paramedic practice can be viewed as the essence of being a team player. Someone who can work alongside anyone, or as an individual, serve as a gatekeeper and, if needed, liaise with relevant healthcare professionals.

and emergency care and rapid response. Though it could be argued that the term paramedic in isolation is sufficient to be identified as first-contact clinical expert.

Do you perceive yourself and the paramedic profession as the expert first-contact clinician? How you perceive yourself as a paramedic is very important. The way in which we demonstrate our collective values and behaviours is shaped by the standards published by our regulator and is included in our curricula and practice guidance. We draw our identity from the training we undertake, sharing values, being members of a professional body and the desire to enhance the standards of paramedic practice. Moving beyond a uniform may incur an identity crisis, yet if you view yourself as an expert first-contact clinician, then this identity ought not to be compromised.

Perhaps, though, it is the public perception of the paramedic role that is the ultimate determinant of the profession's status in society. This is a drastically under-researched area; a recent study in Poland by Majchrowska et al. (2021) randomly surveyed 600 adults, who ranked the paramedic role among other healthcare professionals as one of the most prestigious, and at the forefront of healthcare. This may, however, be a misperceived portrayal based on the media's idea of a paramedic. In addition, not discussed is the multitude of roles paramedics can undertake beyond the clinical realm – academia and education, research, leadership and management – roles that despite being non-patient facing, and arguably definable as non-practising, play an important part in the development of healthcare and the paramedic profession. Future research should explore the public perception of the paramedic role in alternative settings, thus establishing an evidence base that demonstrates how paramedic practice is among one of the most trusted professions at the forefront in Canada.

Decision Making Through the Lens of Bioethics

> *Ethics is nothing else than reverence for life.*
>
> (Albert Schweitzer, 1875–1965)

> *A man without ethics is a wild beast loosed upon this world.*
>
> (Albert Camus, 1913–1960)

Ethics in human healthcare is a vast topic. It covers a wide range of areas and includes very complex models and concepts that have been debated by academics from around the world for centuries. One of the wonders of ethics in particular is the way in which it cross examines human nature, challenging our beliefs as to what is right and wrong, good or bad, and how these concepts fit within varying societies. Most would describe this as morals. Importantly, there is no 'perfect' theory, and many in fact conflict and continue to do so today, even judging the construct of law and society.

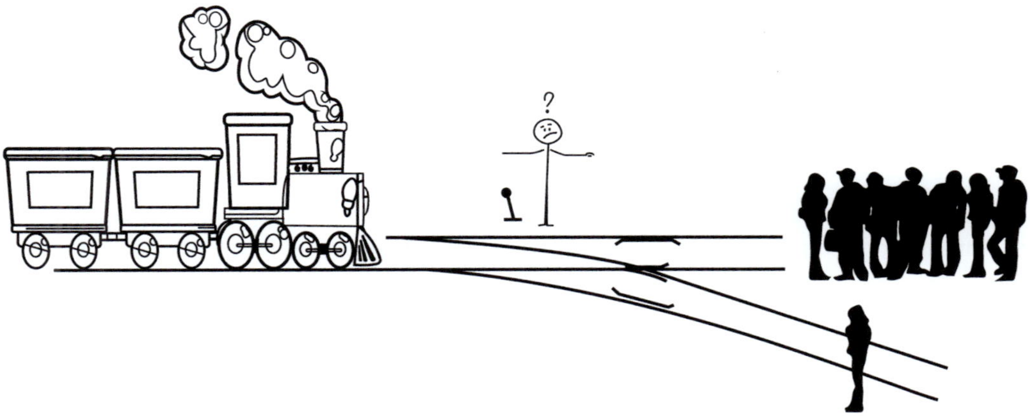

Figure 2.2 The trolley test: A popular thought experiment – to choose to save one or many.

Some great examples of '**thought experiments**' or hypotheticals that explore the complexities of ethics in the healthcare setting include the trolley test[4] (actively switching a lever to save either one person or many where unavoidable harm results – see Figure 2.2) and the rule of rescue.[5] There are simply not enough pages in any book to uncover, explain or present old and new concepts of bioethics; all too often, many pages are dedicated to defining a moral stance or position statement or to explaining existing theories before any attempt is made to delve beyond the basics. As such, this section aims to avoid extensive discussion on generalized ethics, and will focus on how bioethics is symbiotic with any form of decision.

A Brief Overview of Bioethics

There are three main branches of ethics – normative (behaviour, decisions and actions), meta (what does it all mean?) and applied (is it relevant?). For decision making, the main focus is on normative and applied. The two dominant normative theories are the consequentialist theory of **utilitarianism** – 'the greater good' – and **deontology** – 'duty'. Utilitarian thinkers broadly judge actions by considering the outcome, best measured by how much individuals are to benefit with minimal harm to self or others (see the works of Bentham and Mill, the founders, or

[4] Trolley refers notionally to any vehicle on rails that can have its course changed by moving the points from one track to another.

[5] The rule of rescue relates to the desire for individuals, especially paramedics, to place priority on those facing a life-threatening condition, rather than focusing on earlier intervention that stands to serve more benefit in both care and cost. Areas in paramedic practice where this works are heart attacks – earlier recognition and intervention yields improved outcomes, rather than wating for cardiac arrest to occur. Therefore, the rule of rescue argues that sending five paramedics to five patients experiencing heart attacks is more appropriate than five paramedics to a single cardiac arrest (the ambulance dilemma discussed later embellishes on this). Note, that this thought experiment is at risk of marginalizing minority presentations, and there is a balance to be struck between a good prevention strategy (promoting lifestyle during a callout, say), and a reactive one (critical care resources).

more recently, Singer). Deontology, in contrast, focuses on social or universal rules, such as that we ought to behave in a specific manner no matter the outcome. Imagine for instance, you were on the receiving end of the decision about to be made. Would it be acceptable? (See Kant's works – *The Metaphysics of Morals* is a good starting point.) In healthcare, this obligation to act towards others in a reasonable way is known as '**duty of care**'.

Both theories have their strengths and weaknesses. Deontology has constraints and thresholds which, while maintaining integrity, could result in an action causing harm. The classic example is telling the truth about someone's whereabouts when an individual clearly has malicious intent. A healthcare example is breaching confidentiality due to a safeguarding concern or due to a notifiable disease. While a utilitarian would have less of an issue disclosing information to protect others, the fundamental issue with utilitarianism is the benefit or outcome is difficult to measure, which in turn, may render any action justifiable. The aforementioned trolley test is a clear example, but what if that single person was about to discover the cure for cancer, saving countless lives?

An additional branch of ethics that affects decisions is **contractualism**, which reflects the notion of **justice** (equality, fairness and distribution). Who, for example, is entitled to access healthcare and at what cost? *Rawls's Theory of Justice* (1971) dissects this dilemma (particularly against utilitarianism) with a notion called the **'Veil of Ignorance'**. In essence, if we did not know our position in society, would we choose a more equitable one, or would we be accepting of the risk that some people win (e.g., good health or wealth) and some people lose (e.g., disease or poverty) and by how much? This approach is very top down, and Rawls concludes that justice as fairness ought to maximize the worst off in a society (defined as maximin). In contrast, Scanlon (1998) presents a more ground level argument of how we should act based on the circumstance, *with* knowledge of our social position. Are our actions justifiable and reasonable, and could they be mutually agreed upon by others? This in some ways links back to the duty of care.

More recent is the revived proposition of **intuitionism**. This stance contrasts against any claim that an objective moral position can be defined or applied to real world settings. Rather, it contends that moral propositions are self-evident, based on an innate sense of what is a right and good decision that cannot be wholly derived from motive or consequence (Ross, 2002). In other words, when a conflict presents itself, we simply know intuitively what the right action or obligation is (Davis, 2007; Prichard, 1949). If thought about, these self-evident duties can become apparent to some through wisdom and distilled into principles. Ross (2002) thought that duties such as promise keeping, reparation for harm done, gratitude, justice, beneficence, self-improvement and non-maleficence would guide us to do right and good actions. However, he also declared that intuitions are individualistic, and therefore principles may differ between people, societies and cultures. Thus, we cannot truly know whether our actions are right. Despite this contradiction, intuitionism has an important role in triggering our own moral code and demonstrates that through reasoning we can also develop or refine our own obligations and principles.

Nonmaleficence

***Nonmaleficence** means 'first, do no harm'.*

It is accepted that some treatments have associated risks. Paramedics must ensure, therefore, that any treatments considered will provide greater benefit than risk to the patient, and are carried out without malice or other extrinsic reason. The benefits must outweigh the risks, and this is usually supported by clinical guidelines or other evidence-based drivers. Consideration must also be given to the risks of not withholding treatment, as the application of the treatment may also be harmful. For instance, where a patient has chosen not to be resuscitated due to the progression of their terminal illness, CPR is most likely not to be successful. Any injuries (such as rib fractures) caused by CPR will be far more harmful and undignified in the context of trying to prevent the patient's inevitable demise.

Beneficence

A beneficent act is an act that is done for a patient's benefit. Beneficent acts may prevent harm or further harm, and/or can be used to improve the patient's situation.

For paramedics, undertaking resuscitation is the most obvious example of an act of **beneficence**, as carrying out CPR may ultimately prevent death. Beneficence also includes more humanistic acts, such as preserving warmth and dignity, and helping reduce pain.

Beneficence is different from nonmaleficence in that the act moves the patient away from harm and towards an improved situation. Think of it as the difference between pulling someone away from the edge of cliff, compared with pushing them off the cliff into a lake (if the latter was deemed to present less risk of overall harm). In healthcare, encouraging patients to stop smoking or lose weight is a beneficent act as it is intended to prevent harm in the future.

Respect for Autonomy

Respecting autonomy means practising on the basis of the patient's wishes.

Autonomy, or **agency**, is the basic human right which protects the individual's right to self-determination, freedom, will etc. and in healthcare is the basis of patient-centred care. Many patients seen by paramedics have their autonomy suspended or diminished through injury or illness (i.e., head injury or dementia) and this makes decision making harder as, without prior knowledge of the patients' wishes, we may apply our own values and morals to the situation.

Justice

Justice is defined as the fair and equitable allocation of time and resources to promote the correct outcome for patients.

> This concept is of particular interest and should be reflected on by paramedics on the basis that the traditional model of care often bookends patient contact ('one job at a time'). It could be argued that spending three hours with an older person who has fallen and is uninjured, but with whom the paramedic wishes to spend time, may be at the expense of someone with a life-threatening condition waiting longer for a response. The faller gets, in effect, 'too much' justice, and the patient waiting with the life-threatening condition gets less, or no justice. In the context of decision-making, we should consider more carefully how we perceive ourselves as a resource, and how justly we self-allocate this to our patients.

Beauchamp and Childress's (2001) seminal work on healthcare ethics essentially blended the above underlying concepts into 'four principles', or **Principlism**, that help guide any clinician into ensuring that any action is ethically fulfilled if all principles are satisfied. This shifts the ethical lens from the normative to applied domain, since it is used in the real world. The four principles are: beneficence (do good/utilitarian), non-maleficence (no harm/duty), justice (equality, fairness and distribution) and autonomy (self-governing). The last is an adaptation of Kant's (2012) argument that no action should be contrary to the wishes of the person, and importantly prevents clinical paternalism (also known as 'clinician knows best'). These principles aren't without difficulties, particularly when there is a conflict between them, such as when an individual is unconscious, wishes to inflict self-harm or demands (and is willing to pay) for a specific treatment.

Similar to Ross's (2002) intuitionist approach, Beauchamp and Childress (2019) suggest that principles are *prima facie*, 'on the face of things', such that an ethical principle can be diminished should a more pressing obligation be required. In the above examples this would mean diminishing autonomy to balance the other three in helping the individual achieve the best outcome (resolve unconsciousness, prevent further harm to self, reduce unnecessary treatment/access to others). In criticism, the four principles can be broadly misinterpreted to mean anything without a proper understanding of the underlying theory (and to be a little meta-ethical, what does best interests mean in dying?). There is also an argument that the principles themselves are not equally weighted, with autonomy being the fundamental principle to uphold (Gillon, 2015). Indeed, 'do no harm' has existed since Hippocrates (460–370 BC) and may be better placed to guide decisions for those without capacity, such as children (see Diekema, 2019), and the deceased or dying (Dees, 2019) than the other principles.

Lastly and in stark contrast, there is a case for **virtue ethics**, a renaissance theory from ancient philosophers such as Plato, which places focus on an individual being virtuous (based on characteristics such as fidelity, temperance, justice, fortitude and wisdom) and therefore knowing the best course of action in any situation. To be a good, moral person is a fantastic notion to strive towards, and echoes Scanlon (1998). However, little is known on which virtues would make an ideal clinician, how to attain them (it is suggested that this occurs throughout a lifetime), or whether there is generalizability to any given situation or approach in resolving dilemmas (see Banks and Gallagher (2008) for an introduction).

As this section has identified, bioethics is broad and subjective, predominantly theoretical with some overlap between the theories that may or may not be applicable to the real world. Certainly, there is no single 'master' theory, and much of the time ethical positions and stances will change depending on the facing situation. Indeed, when it comes to paramedic practice there are many situations to navigate, from the time-critical through to futile treatments or even deciding when to take a break. The following section focuses on these aspects, developed from the preceding theories, with some evidence to support future models of paramedic bioethical decisions.

Ethical Decision Making in Paramedic Practice

There is some research from around the world that explores or considers how paramedics think ethically. It may be surprising that the overall conclusion is that paramedics focus on beneficence rather than any particular theory or model (Torabi et al., 2019; Davey et al., 2016; Braithwaite, 2014; Nordby and Nøhr, 2012). Although these are small studies that may not be completely generalizable there is a key theme emerging that presents a clear discordance between taught frameworks, such as principlism, and the reality of paramedic practice. Why is this?

The original work of Iserson (1995) illuminates several key issues that differentiates ethics in resource poor environments, such as emergency medicine and pre-hospital care, that are otherwise ignored in the work of Beauchamp and Childress (2019). Focusing on paramedics in the pre-hospital setting, these are:

- Paramedics rarely have a prior relationship with the patient – trust must be gained, lack of choice of clinician, unknown values.
- Time is short.
- The environment is poorly controlled.
- Paramedics have limited clinical support to consult on dilemmas with.

As previously alluded to, these elements do not enable paramedics to deliberate on the minutiae of each decision or action as to whether they are ethical or not. What is emphasized by principlism, such as protecting and acting in the best interests of service users (HCPC, 2016), can cause conflict, confrontation and ethical dilemmas. Consider the notion of Kantian autonomy – freedom to act without internal or external pressure; from the patient perspective much of their autonomy will be dictated by the situation they are in, and their desire to be free from it. This may be an acute illness (such as a thrombotic event), a traumatic incident, self-harm (where the harm itself is an expression of wishing to be freed from a stressor), end of life (the freedom to die with dignity as well as those that do not wish to die), pain, or exacerbation of a chronic disease. In contrast, conflicts of autonomy often arise where the patient is not aware or wanting to be free from the situation. Examples include psychosis, dementia, confusion, intoxication (and this includes overdose), or calls from concerned bystanders (including family members or other healthcare professionals). Finally, autonomy is affected by future situations, such as the perception of going to and waiting in hospital as an inconvenience. Kant's version of autonomy is therefore compromised in patients: a reason why patients are extremely vulnerable to clinician authority and susceptible to over investigation and iatrogenesis.

Example

1. A patient has called at night because they are experiencing severe back pain – they have already made the autonomous decision to call for an ambulance because they feel they can no longer manage the pain and want further assessment (**freedom from pain and underlying cause**).
2. The paramedic arrives and deems it to be a musculoskeletal cause (let's say sciatica). Acetaminophen and ibuprofen are administered, justified as being quick acting, with the option for morphine. Morphine, however, was not given as it was deemed too potent for the amount of relief required. The patient consents (**the patient has consented based on acquiring pain relief despite intravenous access being unnecessary**).
3. The patient is conveyed to hospital overnight and there is limited access to a GP for further analgesia. The advice given is that the hospital will better manage the pain (**pain will be better managed, although there is an increased risk of over investigation**).

The above example demonstrates the complexity of autonomy. There is no perceptible dilemma here, as the patient has consented to each decision. However, the motivation to acquire pain relief results in a sequence of actions between paramedic and patient. The patient has the right to request pain relief, yet the paramedic has the power to decide what and where to give it. How much does the patient understand the risks of intravenous cannulation, and to what extent did they care at that point in time? The rationale to convey yields additional risks and may have been unnecessary, yet was this decision predominantly at the request of the patient or the paramedic?

In contrast to Kantian autonomy, Mill considered autonomy to include the idea of intrinsic self-determination (see *On Liberty*), which is generally more applicable to the real world. However, even this concept of autonomy is not without issue. Consider a dependency on drugs or alcohol. To what extent is a dependent truly self-determined, as in freely choosing to drink alcohol, or are they at the mercy of the substance they crave, unable to abstain? Perhaps then, autonomy needs to be viewed as respecting the wishes of the patient by uncovering their motivations, and also offering a range of options and choices that are provided by the expertise of the paramedic without total authority (paternalism). In essence, sharing the decision. In the above low back pain example, the patient ought to have been offered several choices: the choice to take oral analgesia, or the choice to wait until morning for a GP consultation (the risk being sustained pain). This approach to autonomy results in patient empowerment, fostering an improved self-desire to take control of their situation, and ultimately improves the care they receive (Ubel et al., 2017; Bravo et al., 2015).

Intimately intertwined with autonomy is consent. Kant (2012) rightly suggests that people must be treated as ends in themselves, not a means to an end,[6] meaning that any action cannot be contrary to the wishes of the individual. We can think of consent, then, as the 'signing off' of autonomy (see the Montgomery Rule below). The astute reader and experienced paramedic may be quick to point out that some situations – the unconscious patient, the time-critically unwell, the patient that refuses any suggested plan of action, or those that demand one contrary to advice – are the crux of why the concept of autonomy and consent can be exhausting and stressful.

The Montgomery Rule

The Montgomery Rule introduces the importance of consent in healthcare (*Montgomery v NHS Lanarkshire*, 2015). Consent is a vital aspect of promoting patient-centred care, and even more important in urgent, emergency and unscheduled care, as the patient is more vulnerable and often less able to understand complex concepts due to pain or distress. The Montgomery Rule requires that the clinician ensures the patient understands the seriousness of their condition, any proposed treatments with benefits and risks and ***reasonable alternatives***, so that they are in a position to make an informed decision. The implication of the rule greatly encourages shared decision making. The effective decision maker must of course be decisive, and present a confident front in order for the patient to be reassured as much as possible. Here in Canada, the PERRs CPCF Examination and Education Resources published by COPR and other regulatory documents along with the Paramedic Association of Canada's Canadian Paramedic Profile Code of Ethics include consent as a responsibility to the patient and/or Patient and Community Centered Communication.

In paramedic practice, where autonomous dissent prevails despite offering reasonable alternatives, a paramedic cannot act against an individual's wishes. This is why bioethicists such as Gillon (2015) argue that respecting autonomy is the predominant principle in healthcare. In the absence of autonomy, methods to ascertain the wishes of the patient have been developed, from listening to the patient and their family about their wants and needs, or via pre-agreed documents, such as advanced care planning, to assuming that right to life predominates in the

[6] Kant is notoriously difficult to read, where concepts are typically defined as laws and categorical imperatives. His ideas were highly influential and paved the way for modern (in the western world at least) ethics. Yet, his writing hardly spells out these ideas, resulting in inconsistencies and contradictions. The most famous example is the lack of factoring human emotion in his works, allowing it to be technically impermissible to lie at, say, the risk of another's life. A paramedic instance would be to place one's duty to the care of others over the risk of safety to oneself.

incapacitated until proven otherwise. These situations arguably require a more intuitive approach, such as general and professional moral rules including *'do unto others as you would have them do unto you'* or *'do no harm'*, in order to make either a rapid decision or one that 'best fits' – *prima facie* – as Ross (2002) and Beauchamp and Childress (2019) depict in their writings on intuitionism and principlism, respectively.

Indeed, this may be why studies so far conclude that beneficence is the most prevalent ethical principle among paramedics, as it is more apparent and innate to act in someone's best interests as a healthcare professional than it is to outwardly identify whether patient's needs are concordant with the clinician's decision making. In other words, it is only when disagreement or conflict arises that the autonomy–beneficence relationship is placed under scrutiny. Had existing research accounted for the patient perspective, then it might have become increasingly obvious whether paramedics indeed respect autonomy as much as they serve an individual's

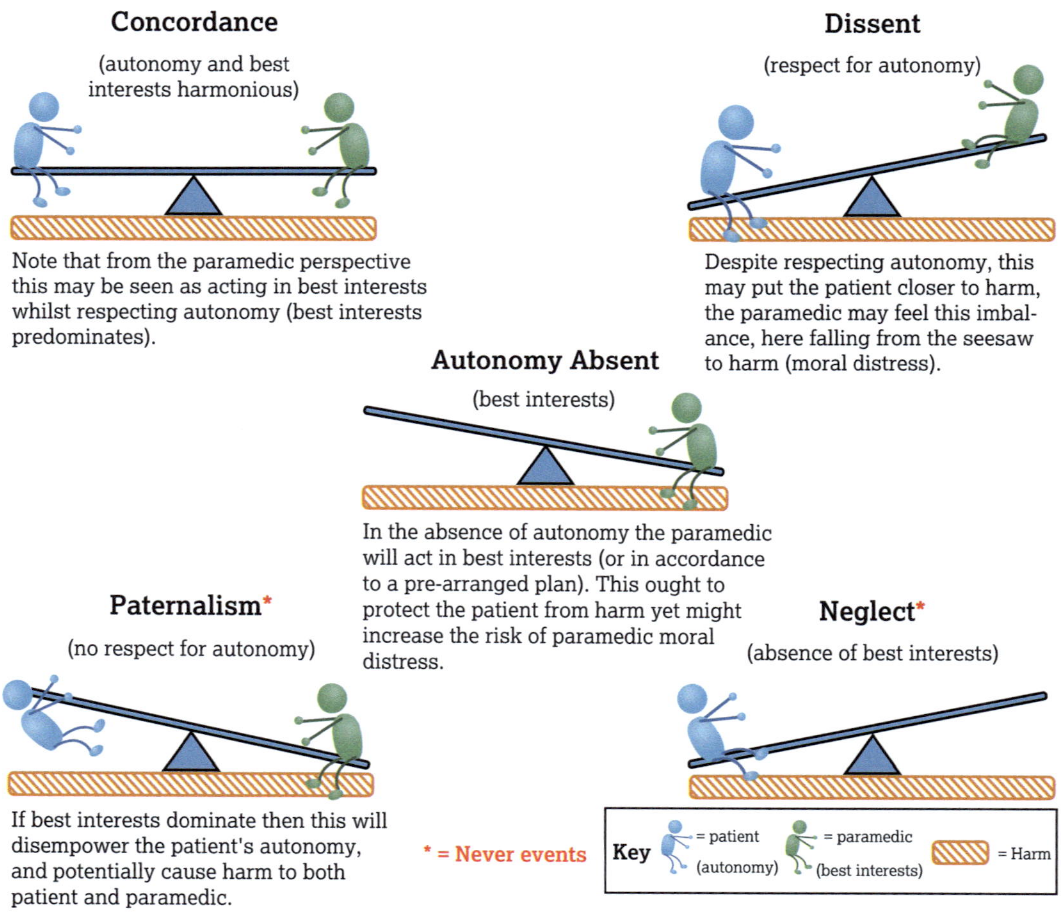

Figure 2.3 The autonomy–beneficence seesaw.
Source: Si Robinson

interests. Thus, we can begin to identify that when we enter into a paramedic–patient relationship, we must acknowledge their autonomy and self-determination, or lack thereof, while acting in the best interests of the patient (see Figure 2.3).

Note how even in paternalism, to the paramedic best interests is predominantly either greater (lower down on the seesaw) or equal to autonomy. In the instance of dissent, this can be distressing to the paramedic.

With Figure 2.3, we can also observe how paramedics might try to avoid causing harm to the patient where possible, maximizing the gap of harm to the patient (the distance of the seesaw to the ground) by making care decisions that minimize risk. As aforementioned, measuring risk is difficult. Certainly, some pre-hospital treatments – thoracotomy, chest compressions, REBOA (resuscitative endovascular balloon occlusion of the aorta) and cricothyroidotomy – are invasive, harmful treatments that seek to save life. Although these treatments are paradoxical to the principle of non-maleficence, the evidential greater benefit versus risk justifies the action. Bear in mind though, that harm extends beyond a physical invasion of the body, which in paramedic practice includes the conveyance of someone to hospital (removal from safe surroundings) as well as over investigation (e.g., excessive blood glucose monitoring); it can also include emotional and social harm. Perhaps the greatest example is dignity in dying, where a paramedic needs to halt further investigation and treatment and manage symptoms which can include drugs at potent doses that would otherwise be harmful to the well (see Blackmore, 2020). In deciding to enact

Doctrine of Double Effect: The Side Effects of Decisions

The doctrine of double effect, introduced by Thomas Aquinas in his discussion of the permissibility of self-defence in *Summa Theologica* (1265–1273, II–II, Qu. 64, Art. 7), argues that causing harm is allowed as a side effect if the intended outcome is a good one. This should not be taken to mean that the end justifies the means (an approach a utilitarian might adopt), but that the overall intention is that of benefit, yet some degree of harm as a consequence unknowingly occurred.

A key example is the administration of a potent dose of morphine at the end of life, of which the intention is to relieve pain, not hasten death. Should death come about as a side effect from this action, then under the doctrine of double effect, this is morally justifiable. However, if the intention was to hasten death as a means to relieve suffering, such as euthanasia, then this would be impermissible. This latter aspect highlights issues with the doctrine of double effect, for if a paramedic foresees that a potent dose of morphine may hasten death rather than relieve pain (rightly or wrongly), then this action may be perceived as more harmful than beneficial. It is therefore important to apply sound ethical judgement, weighing up benefits and risks as well as the wishes of the patient before justifying the action. This could be that the patient is terminally ill, in severe pain and suffering that requires urgent relief, and it could form part of the patient's advanced care plan.

harmful treatments, a paramedic must focus on the overall benefit to the individual, and this can be thought of as the doctrine of double effect.

Beneficence, non-maleficence and respect for autonomy are therefore all intrinsically linked. In many instances, formulating an appropriate care plan with the patient who is in concordance will be an ethically intuitive decision, serving to maximize benefit and minimize harm. But what about contractualism or justice? This notion appears in principlism; however, does it work in synchrony with the other principles, or is it a separate entity that governs principles and decisions in paramedic practice?

Certainly, paramedics owe service to their patients, obliged to help those in need of a paramedic's expertise, in whichever setting a paramedic resides, be it primary, secondary or pre-hospital care. Yet demand far exceeds supply in healthcare, meaning that a single paramedic cannot deal with every individual that requires them. Similarly, a paramedic must use the time with a patient and the resources at their disposal, such as hospital conveyance or requesting additional assistance, wisely. The former elements pertain to distributive justice (Rawlsian), whereas the latter reflects obligation (Kantian and Scanlon).

Regarding obligation, this was introduced earlier in the chapter as the importance of gatekeeping. Is a paramedic obliged to respect the desires of the patient? For instance, if a patient is requesting a treatment that is otherwise unnecessary, ought a paramedic respect their request? Already, this contrasts with respecting the autonomy of the patient: the paramedic has to somehow convince the patient that their self-determination is contrary to their best interests and may even be harmful as a result. Some examples are unnecessary conveyance resulting in over-investigation and increase risk of infection, or the demand for a treatment such as antibiotics (common in primary care). Likewise, to dedicate excessive time to a patient can deprive others in need, a quality potentially deemed as unfair. This latter point is difficult to measure, since good patient care can take time, and who and what type of presentation requires additional attention is hard to define. For the purpose of argument, excessive care can be determined by spending unnecessary time with a patient beyond their needs, by attempting to deliver a treatment that delays onward care (multiple cannulation attempts, for example), or conversely needlessly escalating treatment (such as an inappropriately placing pre-alert calls).

From the conceptual ethical model of the paramedic–patient seesaw, justice can be thought of as the fulcrum, balancing autonomy and interests. If the patient's autonomy 'pushes' the fulcrum against the paramedic's best interests, then autonomy will prevail potentially resulting in harm (this can be represented as requesting treatments). In contrast if the paramedic shifts the fulcrum in favour of the paramedic's interests (and this can be thought of as delivering excessive care, paternalism and coercion, risk aversion, or egoism) then this could resultantly harm the profession by depriving others or breaking down the autonomy–beneficence relationship (see Figure 2.4). The art of maintaining balance stems from a combination of confidence in

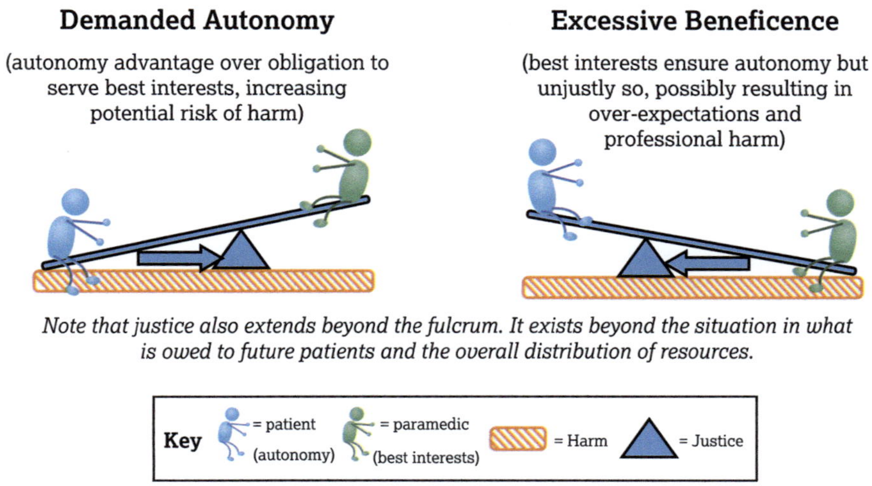

Figure 2.4 The interplay of the four principles.
Source: Si Robinson

practice, professional insight[7] and skilful communication. Note that the onus is on the paramedic, not the patient.

As previously alluded to, justice propagates beyond patient interactions; it is enmeshed in the fabric of our society, which in healthcare generally relates to the distribution and allocation of resources. In paramedic practice, this relates to the number of ambulances available, the access of specialist resources, the types of equipment on the vehicles, and the availability of care pathways. Often, from the ground perspective, there can be frustration that resources are inappropriately used (Phillips, 2020; Dejean et al., 2016; Radcliffe and Heath, 2010). However, understanding the bigger picture of resource distribution can highlight how even with best intentions our actions on the ground yield consequences. The following thought experiment aims to illustrate and challenge moral views on resource distribution.

The Ambulance Resource Problem

Imagine there are three ambulances and three people who have requested an ambulance.

- Person A is in a collapsed state and in cardiac arrest.
- Person B is complaining of slurred speech and thinks it may be a stroke.
- Person C is an older person who has fallen.

[7] Both discussed later in this chapter.

For an optimal resuscitation, person A needs at least two ambulances but may not survive. Person B may, or may not, be having a stroke or require hospital admission (it could be hypoglycaemia), but the facts will not be known until an ambulance arrives on scene. Person C will need admitting if a response and assessment hasn't been made within the hour (rhabdomyolysis concern, for example). Each callout, irrespective of outcome will take an hour to complete (see Figure 2.5).

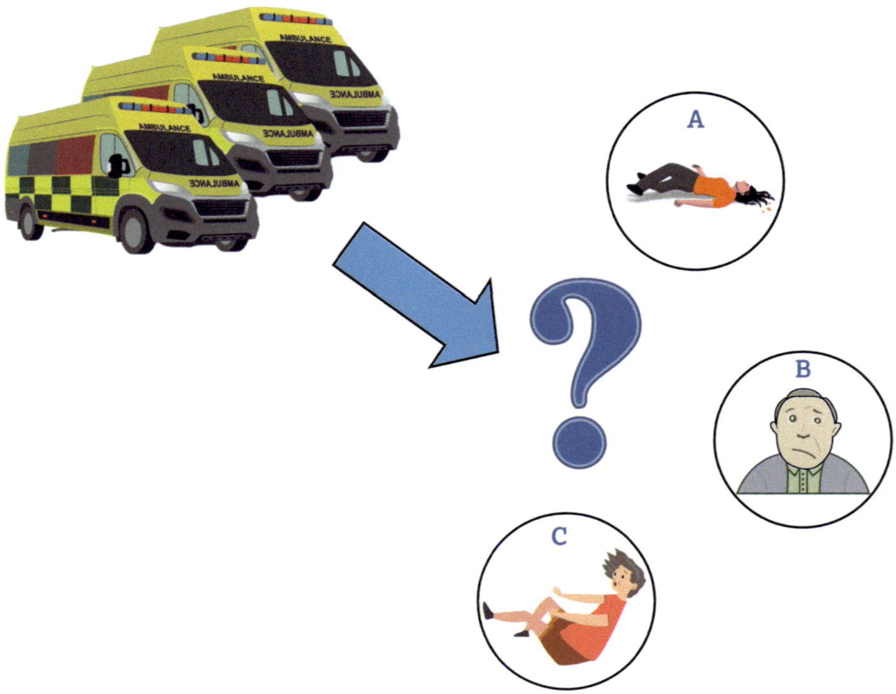

Figure 2.5 The ambulance resource problem.

The problem here is there is no solution without one of the individuals receiving suboptimal care. For example, the simplest solution is the rule of 1/n – distribute the three ambulances equally. That way, Person B and C will have positive outcomes, while person A will receive some degree of care in a likely unsuccessful situation (<10% survival rate). As a paramedic, this may not quite sit right, especially as there is an additional cost to the poor crew delivering extended life support until one of the other ambulances becomes available. Similarly, sending two ambulances to person A means that either person C is guaranteed an admission, or person B will increasingly deteriorate, both of which will cause a greater cost to the wider healthcare system. Nevertheless, person A will be given an optimal chance to survive (but still may not).

The ambulance resource dilemma highlights a conflict between our obligation or duty to help others while maximizing benefit versus risk. The other scenario that causes this dilemma is in mass casualty triage, which according to the ten second triage tool

(NHSE, 2023), adopts a contractualist approach, attempting to prioritize resources. Despite the pragmatism of the tool, it remains open to interpretation: at what point ought a resource be used for CPR (e.g., person A)? It may be somewhere between a priority one (e.g., person C) and a priority two (person B); and if more casualties emerge, is the expectation that a resource ceases CPR to reprioritize? The tool therefore helps focus on specific patients in need, yet might create discrepancies that compels one to act on duty when resources are lacking at a consequence to others.

It is vitally important that paramedics understand that when on the ground managing a patient, it is likely that someone else will be in greater need. This is always the consequence when demand exceeds supply, and as a paramedic you can only possibly manage the patient before you. Fortunately, models and algorithms, such as the Ambulance Response Programme (2017), automate this dilemma and, though imperfect, enable dispatchers and clinicians to sleep better at night. Unfortunately, the dilemma becomes more apparent once paramedics specialize, such as when critical care paramedics self-dispatch to situations, or when community care paramedics decide who receives an appointment or home visit.

Perhaps the simplest solution of 1/n, or first come first served basis resolves such issues, and this circles us back to the intuitionist rule-based argument, where in time-critical, complex situations, a simpler process or mode of thought in the initial phase will likely form an adequate platform for an ethical decision or action. Conversely, where situations are non-complex or low acuity, where there are many more permutations of outcomes, the more critical and reflective we should be of the ethical decision. This is what Einstein meant when he said, '*Everything should be made as simple as possible, but not simpler*' (Einstein, 1933).

Moving Towards a Paramedic Ethical Model

As this section draws to a close, we have identified that the four principles of non-maleficence, beneficence, respect for autonomy and justice do indeed interact in paramedic practice; to avoid harm, the autonomy–beneficence relationship must be recognized, while ensuring that decisions are fair and respectful to the patient's needs and mindful of the resources available. Many decisions will be innately ethical due to the mutual agreement between the paramedic–patient relationship unless a dilemma becomes apparent or reflected upon. Some common dilemmas in paramedic practice identified are:

- Patient dissent with the proposed care plan (autonomy *vs* beneficence).
- Paramedic dissent with the patient's expectations (autonomy *vs* justice/ beneficence).
- Over investigation or delayed care (beneficence/non-maleficence *vs* justice).
- Lack of resources or care pathways (beneficence/non-maleficence *vs* justice).

Resolving dilemmas, however, is more than principles and intuitions alone. It requires critical evaluation of the situation, examining which principles conflict, our moral stance and sense, the limitations and scope of paramedic practice, and failing any obvious solution, an in-depth examination of the underpinning ethical theories to formulate an outcome.

In 1995, Iserson presented a model of rapid ethical decision making that attempted to resolve dilemmas in emergency medicine, including paramedic practice. The model sought to initially reflect on whether a previous rule had been established to inform a decision, say through experience or policy, and if not, to try and 'buy time' without undue harm to the patient, and lastly to consider three tests: impartiality, 'do unto others…'; universalisability, a rule that can be applied to other instances; and justifiability, the action can be justified and defended among other healthcare professionals. Iserson's model, however, has several issues. First, it requires the clinician to recognize that a dilemma is occurring, which in turn promotes rule-based actions rather than considering and balancing principles. Second, not all dilemmas are time-critical, nor do they require time to be bought. Third, the three tests can be crudely interpreted as clinician beneficence rather than any respect for the patient. These oversights may well be due to the time the model was devised, in which both emergency medicine and paramedic practice were in their infancy and tended to focus on the time-critical nature and resource-poor environments that each respective specialty represented and has since evolved from.

In contrast, and not related to either emergency medicine or paramedic practice, Kitchener (1984) devised a model that incorporates both intuitive and critical evaluation of decisions to inform ethical practice among counselling psychologists. The strength of the model is that it reflects the need to identify a problem and act on it in an appropriate manner, both at an immediate, intuitive level and at a higher, evaluative level, incorporating rules and professional codes, principlism, and ethical theory. Although Kitchener did not consider the model for paramedic practice, it closely relates to the preceding argument of how paramedics might approach and resolve a problem ethically. However, the model generally encourages critical reflection as the situation unfolds, which in paramedic practice may not be possible due to time constraints. Further, the model focuses on dilemmas rather than everyday decisions which may in turn have unrecognized ethical issues unbeknown to the paramedic and, indeed, the profession. Therefore, the model below is an adaptation of Kitchener's that focuses on paramedic practice, recognizing both intuitive and critical levels, while encouraging reflection of decisions that are either under time-constraint or seemingly innocuous.

The Paramedic Ethical Decision-making Model

The paramedic ethical decision-making model (see Figure 2.6) also closely aligns with clinical decision-making models, as the rest of this book will uncover. It is important to remember, though, like much of ethics, the model remains theoretical, and despite the argument set out in this chapter, requires research to further evidence whether paramedics indeed think beyond intuition and best interests alone.

Indeed, in his book *Against Bioethics* Jonathan Baron makes an interesting observation, which illustrates this point very effectively: '. . . many moral intuitions are interesting psychological phenomena rather than windows into some sort of moral truth' (Baron, 2006: Preface, P xi).

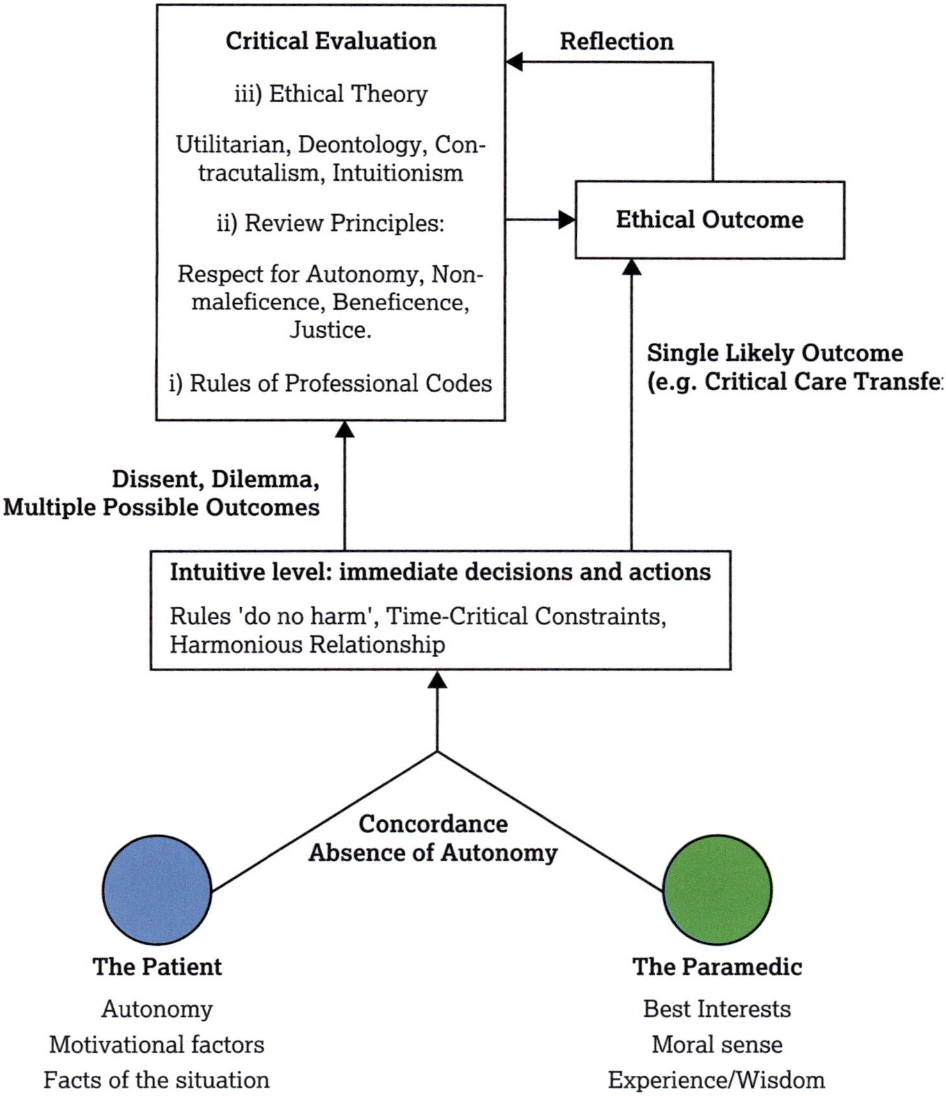

Figure 2.6 The paramedic ethical decision-making model.
Source: Si Robinson

This section has barely scratched the surface of ethics, but there is a wealth of literature available, and the books and journal articles referenced in the text and listed in the Further Reading section at the end of this chapter should provide a useful start for further reading. A good place to start is Eaton's (2024) book *Law and Ethics for Paramedics*.

Patient-centred Care

In Canada patients quite correctly have a voice, and this voice is aimed both at the shaping of services and at defining how healthcare encounters happen. In days gone by, healthcare was done to patients, rather than with them, and concepts such as shared decision making and patient empowerment were not yet considered.

Comedy films from the 1960s and 1970s with a healthcare theme such as some of the Carry On series and Doctor in the House depicted the often paternalist nature of hospital-based care in that era. An example of this is a scene in the 1967 film *Carry on Doctor*, which shows actor Jim Dale forcibly having his underwear removed by a rather domineering nurse, played by the actress Hattie Jacques. Although comedic, the response from the patient typifies the importance of communication and consent. In biomedical ethics, the patient is paramount with Kantian, duty-based ethics stating that patients 'must always be the end in themselves and never a means to an end' (Kant, translated Bennett, 2008). In emergency care, and as paramedic practice has developed, the issue of consent has become ever more complex but increasingly better defined. The combination of an action-biased workforce and the notion of 'presumed consent' has led the need to move the patient to the centre, and ensure that they are fully informed of their care. Patients are also extremely useful for decision makers, and quite apart from the ethical and value-based imperative, they often hold the key to their own illness or injury. History taking accounts for 90–95% of the diagnostic process, and while some warn of the 'bad historian', the clinician should apply competent processes that prevent the patient from failing to express their condition and impede a good diagnosis.

> *Listen to your patient, he is telling you the diagnosis.*
>
> (Sir William Osler, 1849–1919)

Consent is important in urgent, emergency and unscheduled care, as the patient is more vulnerable and often less able to understand complex concepts due to pain or distress. The effective decision maker must of course be decisive and present a confident front in order for the patient to be reassured as much as possible. But the balance must be struck between rote, paternalistic care delivery and care that is delivered in partnership with the patient, and wherever possible that care is delivered with the full informed consent, or at least assent, of the patient. Patient-centred care is much more than a modern buzzword in healthcare, and can be considered in the following analogy.

A woman takes her car to the local garage complaining that the car is making a funny noise. She says she thinks the exhaust has a hole in it. 'Of course it's got a hole in it, that's where the fumes come out!' the mechanic says. 'No, a new hole. It's making a rasping noise, and I need some advice.' The mechanic explains that he can change the exhaust if she would like. The woman isn't a mechanic and does not have the expertise to know whether the exhaust can be repaired. She is worried that this might be an unnecessary expense, and the experience is making her anxious and upset. Imagine if that was in a healthcare encounter. The woman knows that something is wrong and it might be simple and easy to treat. In the case above, had the mechanic used the equivalent of patient-centred care, the scenario would have been very different. How many times have you seen a patient's needs dismissed because the patient wasn't put first, perhaps because they couldn't express their concerns?

Remember, the patient must only ever be the end, and never a means to an end. Another example, seen in Chapter 1, was that of the paramedics who took a patient to hospital, despite the fact that the patient clearly could have been cared for in the community, because they knew they could get themselves a cup of tea at the hospital. The patient is paramount. The patient's experience of care often affects their outcome and recovery. Always base your decision making about the patient on what is best for them.

Confidentiality: The Crossroads Between Professionalism and Bioethics

This chapter has discussed the importance of patient trust through professional behaviour and regulation, as well as the importance of respecting autonomy from a self-determined sense while maintaining the balance of best interests and justice. Betraying these elements not only causes harm to the patient but also the profession. There is no greater instance that represents the clinician–patient bond than that of confidentiality. Patients' personal information must be protected and yet there are very limited circumstances where not respecting a patient's confidentiality can be considered, such as protecting others from infectious diseases or where a crime has been committed. Thus, we have met a juncture that connects professionalism and bioethics with the decisions we make.

Here in Canada the privacy of health information requires a familiarity with both federal and provincial law. Some provinces choose to adopt federal privacy laws in which paramedics must be familiar with in their practice. There are also provinces such as Nova Scotia, Ontaio and Newfoundland that have provincial laws such as the Personal Health Information Protection Act in Ontario that apply to paramedic practice. Maintaining confidentiality is an active process. Clinicians should include, within their decision-making process, the steps they will consider to protect patients' data.

There are still many pitfalls, which may not be considered directly by paramedics in practice, the most common one being the use of social media.

The use of social media by healthcare professionals to support CPD and intercollegiate communication is growing, and this can be very positive. However, there is also a rise in the practice of recording and sharing experiences through these platforms as an extension of healthcare professionals' private lives. The decision-making processes used in diagnosis and patient management can be applied to choices regarding social media. For example, the decision to photograph the scene of a road accident and post to social media may provide a point of interest for friends and family. Not only might this be tasteless and inappropriate on both a personal and professional basis, but also if a patient is identified as a result of this, or information is deemed to have been shared inappropriately or otherwise in line with the responsibilities of the registrant, the consequences may be significant. Sanctions have been applied in several cases in recent years.

Competence and Confidence in Practice

The theme, which appears throughout this book, is the link between competency and confidence in practice, linked to the need to practise defensibly (rather than defensively – see Chapter 7). Let's consider the definition of confidence in the context of clinical practice – as opposed to keeping secrets!

> **Competency**: '*an important skill that is needed to do a job.*'
>
> **Confidence**: '*the quality of being certain of your abilities or of having trust in people, plans, or the future.*'
>
> (Cambridge Dictionary, 2017)

Unlike confidence, competency can be viewed as qualitative, as well as quantitative. The acquisition of skills may be binary (able or unable to) and can be assessed accordingly as evidence of ability. Alternatively, it may emerge over a period of time along a 'novice to expert' path. Can we assess confidence in the same way? How can we remind ourselves that we either are confident, or should be confident?

Confidence is a lived experience, and is a psychological condition, which is hard to assess compared to psychomotor skills (**suturing**, for instance). It may be felt by the individual and/or observed by others, for instance:

- After that last resus, she has really lost her confidence.
- I have never been confident when dealing with children.
- Passing the exam really improved my confidence.

Being confident has a positive impact on patients, and no patient wants to be cared for by a healthcare professional who lacks confidence and displays this outwardly. Confidence in practice may be linked to culture, local policy, management style or a host of other issues, which may be directly or indirectly linked to clinical practice. Approaching problems with confidence is important, and learning what you can be confident about is a way of overcoming the anxieties that can impact negatively on your time in the workplace. The notion of **epistemological** self-confidence – a belief in what you know and what you do – is certainly something to aim for if you are starting from a position of weak confidence. It is certainly preferable to over-confidence or complacency.

Confidence in practice grows over time but can also diminish following events and the risk of a poor outcome. Confidence can be optimized through reflection, self-awareness, consolidated experience, and willingness to learn from error. Healthcare is developing a more just culture in which learning can drive continuous improvements in care. Building and maintaining confidence is on a gradient, which may differ depending on the type of patient you are seeing (trauma *vs* medical, for example). Ultimately, though, confidence colours your experience in practice, and so should be seen as something to work on and develop in the same way you develop your other skills.

Professional Insight

In Chapters 3 and 4, we will discuss some of the biases and fallacies that beset the human condition, such as the issue of unconscious incompetence (I don't know what I don't know). This in turn links closely to professional insight: knowing what you know about yourself and how this may affect the care you give. It is subtly different from technical competence and is associated with more complex considerations, including the ego, which impacts on how you feel and function. Conditioning yourself to have a healthy scepticism of your own ability is vitally important (see 'Mount Stupid' in Chapter 5, p. 127) and will work to support your practice and protect your patient.

Insight is defined as awareness and perception, understanding and comprehension, and perspicacity, and infers a deep cognitive view on how things really are. An astute self-assessment of how well you perform can lead to far better decisions and should be seen in a very positive (rather than a defeatist) way. This can inform how delegation takes place at the patient's side – you may assess your own ability to achieve difficult IV access in comparison to a colleague who has previously demonstrated to you that they are more proficient, and therefore more likely to succeed. Parking your own ego and focusing on the logical argument can provide a greater sense of achievement in how ultimately care is delivered. This requires professional insight and, to some degree, personal sacrifice.

Professional insight has a very real utility in the presence of error and harm, and how you behave and respond to situations that have a poor outcome. Those with strong professional insight are the first to raise their hand where things go wrong and are less likely to cover up their mistakes, choosing instead to learn from them. Where professional insight is strongest, the decision to share the event with colleagues in an action learning group or peer review may happen.

Conclusion

Professional practice extends beyond the confines of the patient–clinician interface, and the acts, omissions, judgements and behaviours of all healthcare professionals must be considered in the context of your professional identity and standards. Registered healthcare practice also extends beyond periods of time at work, and while this may appear overbearing, it is a reflection of the trust and faith society has on those with the skills and aptitude to provide care for patients. Paramedics often provide care for patients when their needs are at the most acute, and sometimes during situations where the environment is at its most hostile – such as the terrain, the weather or even hostile people.

Professional considerations are unlikely to be explicitly included in guidelines and protocols and can exist in the murky areas between best practice, legislation, humanity and morality. Navigating professional issues can be made clearer through the decision you make if you take a moment to consider these in the context of the practice dilemma being managed. Your developing decision-making skills will help you maintain patient safety and will prompt you to think critically rather than accept what you may have unknowingly processed in the past.

The end of this chapter concludes the concepts and principles that together can form a model for you to use and develop in practice in order to make safe, ethical and defensible decisions for your clinical encounters with your patients. As with many things in life, the processes described are theoretical and represent only a modicum of the perspective of how and why humans (in this case paramedics) make decisions. There are many ways to achieve the goal of becoming an effective decision maker, and you may want to keep reading perhaps more deeply into the field of sociology, ethics or psychology and determine your own perspective and even ultimately challenge the ones written here, since this is how as a profession, we can continue to advance the field of paramedic practice and decision making. Thus, the purpose of this whole book is to open up lines of enquiry within oneself in order to face the main issue that befalls human beings who are asked to do complex tasks: we weren't designed to do any of this! The constant conflict between the quick, impulsive and overall less tiresome part of ourselves that effortlessly makes decisions (thought to be our base ancestral heritage 'old brain') and the more thoughtful, deliberate part, which can be exhausting, is what causes bad decisions and bad outcomes, not to mention all the additional factors including emotion, fatigue and empathy that contribute to errors in judgement. It can be improved upon by using techniques that encourage you to challenge and reflect on your everyday experiences.

The days of using only experience and intuition, with the safety net of being able to move patients to another professional or care setting every time, are over. Many patients have manageable presentations in the community, and the way decisions are made needs to be done with a wider range of cues and considerations. These considerations must be analysed critically – sometimes using scepticism and cynicism – but always focused on doing the right thing. The next chapter will look in more detail at critical thinking as a foundation for approaching and managing challenges in practice.

Reflective Exercises

1. What is unique about being a paramedic? Can you identify specific aspects that the paramedic profession has that make it attractive and versatile to a multitude of settings? Could this limit or enhance decision making among other professions?
2. Ethical considerations are extremely important for patients in clinical practice. Are you able to identify your natural ethical stance (for instance, intuitionist, utilitarian, justice as fairness, deontologist) and see how it might affect how you think about situations where there is a conflict? Using bioethics and the interplay of the four principles, can you apply them to a case you have dealt with and determine how your stance and knowledge of the principles influenced your decision making and the outcome?
3. Consider the importance of professional insight in your own practice. Test your own levels of humility and ego, reflecting on errors you have made in the past. How can your insight drive improvements to your knowledge and skill without diminishing your confidence?
4. Select one of the published regulatory standards documents from the COPR website. Reflect on the importance of it in relation to the function of the regulator. Why is this important, and what do paramedics need to understand as an intrinsic aspect of their practice?

Further Reading

Below is a small selection of books that bear relevance to the ethics and professionalism of paramedic practice that might open up an internal discourse and pave a way for further intrigue in the subject.

Beauchamp, T.L. and Childress, J.F. (2001) *Principles of Biomedical Ethics*. Oxford: Oxford University Press.

Arguably the book that defines bioethics and principlism, it is comprehensive in defining the four principles and developing an argument for the applicability for them. A long read and not always relatable to paramedic practice.

Campbell, A. (2017) *Bioethics: the basics*. Abingdon: Routledge.

A broad overview of ethics in healthcare with differing moral theories and perspectives as well as some classic clinical examples that healthcare professionals are confronted with. A short read.

Clarke, A. (2013) *The Sociology of Healthcare*. Abingdon: Routledge.

A comprehensive volume covering aspects of professionalism and identity, as well as patient groups and theories on health.

Eaton, G. (2022) *Law and Ethics for Paramedics*. 2nd Edn. Bridgwater: Class Professional Publishing.

Specifically for paramedics, discussing the frequent confrontations paramedics encounter including topics on end of life, children, mental health, organ donation and research. Moderate read, useful as reference to relevant chapters.

Iserson, K., Sanders, A., and Mathieu, D. (1995) *Ethics in Emergency Medicine*. Tuscon: Galen Press.

Although dated, this book addresses ethical dilemmas in resource poor and time critical settings, with sections dedicated to paramedics. It is important to note this refers to North American paramedic practice with notable differences in the justification of best interests and the law (and regulation). It does, however, highlight how to be an effective quick thinker.

Chapter 3

Decision-making Theory: Dilemmas and Conundrums

Si Robinson and Andy Collen

Chapter Objectives

This chapter will cover:

- Models of reasoning
- The hypothetico-deductive model
- Heuristics – pattern recognition
- Dual process theory
- Naturalistic decision making
- The cognitive continuum
- Patient safety – error, blame and just culture
- Checklists and structured communication
- Human fallibility and biased thinking – learn before you make mistakes.

Introduction

Each and every day we make decisions; some are trivial, such as deciding to have a cup of tea or what to eat for dinner, and some are complex, for example planning a family or purchasing a house. Often, however, these decisions directly involve and affect us, where we have complete access to our innermost thoughts, past experiences and, to a degree, our knowledge. Yet as healthcare professionals, much of our professional decisions will affect others, most of all our patients, who trust that through our expertise we will make a decision that betters their life.

There are three main categories of decisions made for patients by paramedics. These are:

- Diagnostic decisions – assessing, testing, clinical impressions, diagnosing.
- Treatment decisions – medication administration, splinting, reassuring.
- Management decisions – explaining, advising, referring, safety netting.

There is a degree of overlap and consequence between these types of decisions. For instance, an inaccurate diagnostic impression can lead to an error in treatment or management. Furthermore, as a paramedic specializes, the risk of error within a decision category increases. In critical care, this may be a treatment decision, such as thoracostomy or cardioversion. In urgent care, it could be advising a poor management strategy. An expert decision maker will utilize a combination of knowledge and experience to minimize the chance of error with maximum efficiency.

How, though, do we make decisions? And how is error minimized efficiently?

The following chapter explores some cogent theories that are used in healthcare to make a reasoned decision, highlighting the benefits and pitfalls posited by each theory, and discussing when and how it is appropriate to adopt a certain approach in practice.

Before proceeding, it would be wise to highlight some golden rules of paramedic practice, as it would be unrealistic to expect any clinician to always make perfect decisions without error based on the above three categories. Remember these golden rules:

1. Diagnostic certainty is rare – this is especially the case in unscheduled and resource-poor settings. It could take weeks or months, multiple tests and trial medication to reach a more formal conclusion.
2. It is better to rule out than rule in – excluding life-threatening conditions is more important than figuring out the underlying disease.
3. Some risk is inevitable – understanding how to mitigate deterioration and how to safety net is arguably more important than any decision itself (see Chapter 6).
4. Knowing the outcome of the decision might not improve future decisions – perhaps a controversial point, and one discussed in more detail in Chapter 6. However, it is important to understand that feedback can introduce bias, particularly when considering points 1 and 2.

These rules fall under the realms of **normative decision theory.** This is not to be confused with normative ethics, but is in fact a very close relative. Normative decision theory focuses on what an individual ought to choose when faced with a decision problem (Elliot, 2019). These decisions are thought to be constructed from logic and rationality. However, the works of Kahneman and Tversky in the 1970s, which led to influential publications (Kahneman and Tversky, 1979), illustrated that in reality, behaviour is also a significant component that causes individuals to (predictably) deviate from a decision that would otherwise seem logical. This falls under the branch of **descriptive decision theory**, which explores what people actually do when making a decision.

Perhaps you read the golden rules and instantly disagreed with them, with thoughts such as *'I know what a STEMI looks like'* or *'feedback will make me a better clinician'* or *'paramedic practice isn't black and white'*, which are all valid arguments that illustrate the divisiveness of how we apply our knowledge, experience and emotion to decisions, and how theories and models can fail to encapsulate (or agree) on how these decisions come about. As this chapter unfolds, we shall see that there are many ways to reach a decision.

Models of Reasoning

Much of any formal training in healthcare involves hours of learning anatomy and pathophysiology, and developing an understanding of the signs and symptoms that indicate a certain disease. This acquired knowledge enables a logical argument that derives a premise that needs to be reasoned with before establishing a conclusion. In the instance of decision making, this may be a proposition such as a diagnosis (or clinical impression) that can then be actioned upon by way of a management plan.

In a nutshell, a paramedic sees a patient, information is gathered in the form of visual cues and history taking, knowledge and experience are then used to present a logical argument that is thought through (reasoned), to which a rational conclusion is advised. Remember golden rule #2 means that the conclusion does not need to be a confirmation; it is perfectly acceptable to reason what conditions are unlikely and refer on to a more senior clinician.

There are many types of reasoning. The two most common examples are deductive and inductive reasoning, yet many other reasoning methods have a useful role in clinical practice. The following section introduces types of reasoning that are applicable to paramedic decision-making.

Deductive Reasoning

Simply put, deductive reasoning is the application of general scientific principles to a particular case (Brush, 2015) (Figure 3.1). Logically, the truth of a principle or premise guarantees the truth of the conclusion. The advantage of deductive thinking is the absolute certainty that if the premise is true, the conclusion is true.

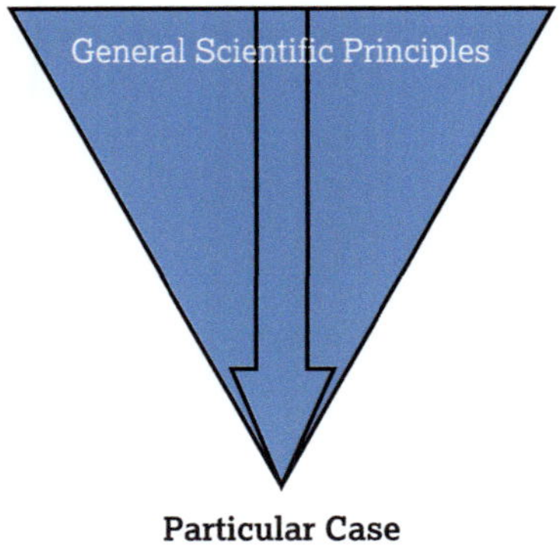

Figure 3.1 Deductive reasoning.

The following are examples of deductive reasoning.

Premise: Hypoglycaemia presents with low capillary blood glucose <4.0 mmol/L.

My patient Pat has a blood glucose 3.0 mmol/L.

Conclusion: Pat is hypoglycaemic.

Premise: Sudden acute onset of chest pain after exertion should have an ECG as part of the assessment.

My patient Jude has acute chest pain.

Conclusion: An ECG needs to be undertaken.

However, deduction is only as accurate as the validity of the premise. The truthfulness of the premise may be affected by errors of knowledge, a lack of evidence or atypical presentations. You may have even heard the adages: 'nothing ever presents like the textbook' and 'presentations are never black and white'. Indeed, deductive reasoning is poor at predicting future events, and in healthcare it is seldom used in isolation due to the risk of going very wrong if the premise is not textbook.

Premise: Excessive insulin can cause hypoglycaemia in diabetics.

My patient Pat is hypoglycaemic.

Conclusion: Pat must be a diabetic who used too much insulin.

While the premise is true, Pat may be hypoglycaemic from other causes, such as fasting, alcohol, infection or exercise. It may not even be related to diabetes!

Inductive Reasoning

In opposition to deduction, inductive reasoning uses evidence through specific investigation to derive a more general conclusion. Typically, a pattern of signs and symptoms are grouped to help rationalize what the underlying disease might be (Figure 3.2). Inductive reasoning is commonplace in healthcare (Hughes and Nimmo, 2016), and paramedicine is no exception.

However, inductive reasoning cannot guarantee a conclusion, only a probable one. The British philosopher, David Hume (1711–1776) wrote in his *Treatise of Human Nature* that 'instances of which we have had no experience resemble those of which we have had experience' (Book I, Part III, Section VI). For example, a patient suffering from a myocardial infarction, does not imply that the following patient with matching

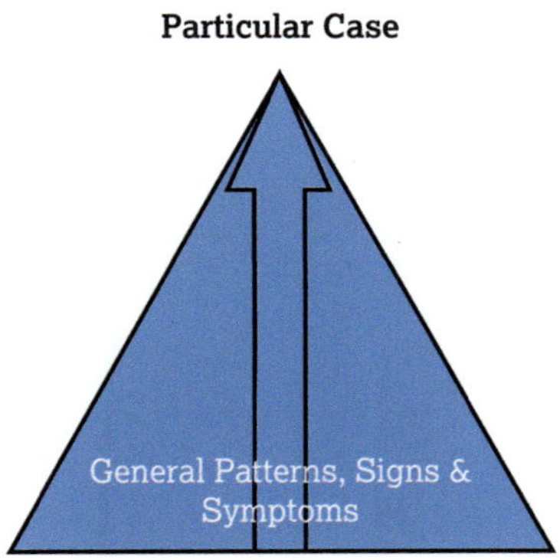

Figure 3.2 Inductive reasoning.

patterns, is also experiencing a myocardial infarction. It might be a severe case of pericarditis, pulmonary embolism, aortic dissection, or related to cocaine use. This ties in with golden rules #1 and #4 – it is reasonable to expect a condition to be present based on a thorough assessment or specific set of patterns, and therefore treat accordingly; however, be mindful that it could be something else entirely!

Here are some examples.

Premise: Robin is presenting with FAST positive symptoms (facial or limb weakness, or slurred speech). There is no history of alcohol or hypoglycaemia.

Conclusion: Robin is possibly experiencing an acute stroke – note that until further tests are undertaken, such as a CT scan, we have no idea if this is the case, or if it is, which type it might be.

Premise: Francis is complaining of dysuria, increasing urgency and frequency with some mild flank pain.

Conclusion: Francis is suspected to have a urinary tract infection. It may well be upper, lower, psychogenic or some other renal pathology. It would be worth treating as such with some further investigation, such as urinalysis and sending a sample to the laboratory (in primary care), but highlighting concerns should symptoms persist or alter.

Abductive Reasoning

The simplest way to explain abductive reasoning is that it is the 'most plausible explanation'. Although it is not particularly cited in paramedic literature, it is commonly used. The rationale for abductive reasoning is when an incomplete picture is formed, either through lack of access to diagnostic tests or history, and the decision has to rely on a pragmatic blend of inductive and deductive thinking.

Premise: A person lies unconscious in the street right outside the pub. It is New Year's Eve. An empty bottle of beer is next to them, and their vital signs are unremarkable.

Conclusion: The incident is likely to be alcohol related.

Premise: A 58-year-old man is in witnessed cardiac arrest, last seen clutching his chest with an initial rhythm of ventricular fibrillation.

Conclusion: The cause of cardiac arrest is highly likely to be an acute myocardial infarction.

Abductive reasoning can infringe on golden rule #2, and so it is important to rule out other more serious causes before actioning a decision.

Causal Reasoning

The academics will always chime that 'correlation does not imply causation', which in research means that variables are related somehow yet it is difficult to deduce cause and effect. In clinical practice, causal reasoning is a vital element of confirming how a disease came about.

Premise: Alex has smoked a pack of cigarettes every day for the past 40 years and is now short of breath on exertion. No other symptoms are present.

Conclusion: Chronic obstructive pulmonary disease is the most likely diagnosis, although smoking increases the risk of other pathology, which would need to be further discussed with a senior clinician.

Premise: Frankie fell off their bicycle after hitting the curb, landing on their shoulder, which now hurts. There are no other injuries or symptoms.

Conclusion: Acute trauma to the shoulder is the most likely cause of the pain.

According to Kassirer et al. (2010), causal reasoning is considered more of a cognitive ingredient to aid decisions, to which there are three components to the causal framework:

1. A causal field – a context in which reasoning about probable cause occurs (the example of long-term smoking or road traffic collisions).
2. Cues to a relationship – the evidence that certain elements have a relationship (smoking and lung disease, falling and injuries).

3. Factors that influence causal strength – whether all signs point towards the presenting complaint or to the contrary; as per golden rule #2, whether alternatives are equally or more likely.

The Hypothetico-deductive Model

The hypothetico-deductive model is an influential framework of clinical decision making originally devised by Elstein et al. (1978). The title of the model is somewhat of a misnomer, as it incorporates both inductive and deductive reasoning methods to confirm or refute a hypothesis from a range of differentials that is generated by the clinician. From here more refined models merge, such as the four stages system outlined by Radwin (1990):

1. Cue acquisition – information seeking such as history taking and overall presentation.
2. Hypothesis generation – considering a range of possibilities.
3. Cue interpretation – refining by seeking further tests or focused questions.
4. Hypothesis evaluation – favouring a management decision based on the evidence.

The benefits of such a structured approach are that it offers the clinician a chance to consider a range of possibilities and exclude them (golden rule #2!) towards a working diagnosis. It also acts as a strategy to think before acting, ensuring that mismanagement is minimal. However, the model itself is limited by the same boundaries discussed in both inductive and deductive reasoning. That is, a paramedic's range of differentials will depend on pre-existing knowledge and that it can never be said for certain that a disease is present.

Case example

A 45-year-old woman presents with an urticarial rash on her trunk that she noticed about an hour ago. It is itchy. She has no known allergies or medical history, and the last thing she remembers eating was a salad for lunch. She has called an ambulance because she feels she is having a serious allergic reaction.

Your examination reveals no further symptoms, and her basic vital signs are unremarkable.

Using the hypothetico-deductive model, write down some differentials and think up some further questions.

On further questioning she states that this has never happened before, and reports no history of being bitten by animals or insects. She has not tried any herbal remedies or medications, and does not smoke or drink. In fact, she has recently become vegan after being a vegetarian for the past two years. There is no significant family history. Socially, she lives with her partner, who is well, she is not pregnant, has no pets and works in an office. Her home appears tidy. To reiterate, she has no fever, and any further pre-hospital test is unremarkable.

Of your hypotheses, which is your preferred choice? What is your treatment (if any) and management plan?

Now reflect on how confident you are with this decision; if you aren't, that's okay.

What you should have concluded is that this rash is unlikely to be life-threatening, and while you might be unsure what it is, the patient doesn't need to go to the emergency department. If you decided to administer an antihistamine, this may have helped but would not have treated the underlying cause. The model answer would have been to discuss with her GP and arrange further investigations, such as a blood test.

You earn bonus points if you placed vitamin deficiency, thyroid disease, dietary and idiopathic causes on the differentials list, the most likely culprit being vitamin deficiency (iron).

As the example case illustrates, the hypothetico-deductive method is a slow, deliberate process, limited to clinician knowledge and the ability to gather an accurate history. It can be mentally exhausting and susceptible to cognitive overload that, when under pressure in time-critical situations or complex presentations such as multi-morbid elderly people, can lead the clinician to make significant errors.

Heuristics – Pattern Recognition

There is a reason why the primary survey and the initiation of basic life support is drummed into a paramedic-to-be from day one; these cognitive actions become embedded and start to feel so natural that actually explaining how they are enacted is often harder than simply just performing them. This is an example of **heuristic** thinking.

Heuristics are learned mental processes that help us to rapidly solve uncertain, unstructured problems (Brush, 2015). A more colloquial way of explaining heuristics is that they are 'rules of thumb', a combination of pattern recognition, fast mental checklists, trial and error, and anchoring and adjusting. For instance, look at Figure 3.3.

You likely did not think twice in determining that the rhythm is ventricular fibrillation (pattern recognition), and quicker still, you knew exactly what to do next and may not have even flinched in reaching for a shock button (fast mental checklists)!

Heuristics have been mentioned in the previous chapter, and the ability to think quickly is important in paramedic practice, particularly for time-critical rapid decisions that prevent harmful delay. However, heuristics can also be subject to biased thinking (Kahneman, 2012). For example, in the earlier example of urticaria

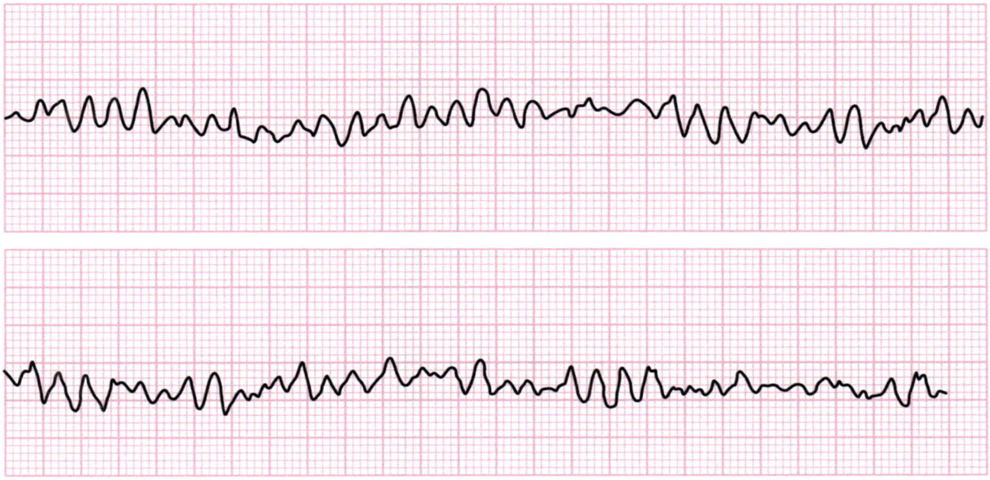

Figure 3.3 ECG showing ventricular fibrillation.

the woman was concerned she was having an allergic reaction. This may have led to a bias due to the fact that urticaria can be associated with an allergic reaction, therefore causing the decision narrative to reach for what seems a salient or representative solution.

The application of 'rules of thumb', or indeed the golden rules presented within this chapter, are a heuristic that can counterbalance bias. Gigerenzer (2015) argues that by simplifying, we can filter out excess information or processes, which can lead to better decision making. Even Kahneman (2012), to a degree, agrees with this. Nevertheless, knowing which rules are simple enough to make a good decision relies on expert experience and evidence. An individual who looks unwell – cyanosed, dyspnoeic, clammy and diaphoretic – presents a pattern that conforms within the primary survey to an escalation of care being required. In contrast, a wheezy infant who is playful and otherwise well may result in a less confident decision without first seeking further action, such as asking questions and checking vital signs; yet the final decision (advising watchful care and GP involvement) is very likely to be the same. Hence, heuristics play an important role in recognizing when to be concerned and conduct more tests and treatment, and when to be reassured that further investigation is unlikely to yield a change in outcome. Importantly, good application of heuristic thinking is a sign of an expert.

However, poor heuristics can and will lead to poor decisions, bias and potentially harmful action. The following are some examples of poor 'rules of thumb' in paramedic practice:

- 'If in doubt, convey the patient to hospital' (excessive testing, waste of resources).
- 'Don't ever forget blood glucose' (excessive testing).

- 'If this isn't acted on now, an adverse event will happen' (risk aversion).
- 'If you hear hoofbeats, think of horses, not zebras' (the equivalent of ruling in – you WILL miss the zebra when it comes).

Dual Process Theory

The dual process theory puts forward the view that our thoughts, and subsequently our decisions, can emerge in two different ways – often through an implicit or heuristic process, as well as through an explicit or more conscious process. In essence, dual process theory combines the hypothetico-deductive model with heuristics, such that heuristics act as the 'spark plug' in our **cognition** to which we then either switch to more detailed thought processes or continue intuitively.

Neuroscience and psychological research have revealed that our brains will take short cuts when decision making by categorizing and forming preferences. Daniel Kahneman, the psychologist who has researched decision making and judgement, concluded that the brain uses two systems for judgement and decision making. Kahneman named these System 1 and System 2 (Kahneman, 2012):

- System 1: Judgement and decision making is rapid, based on intuition and emotion.
- System 2: Judgement and decision making is slower, based on problem solving and deliberate, logical thinking.

Kahneman (2012), to whom we'll refer throughout this book, popularized this concept of System 1 (intuition/heuristic) and System 2 (deliberate thought/hypothetico-deductive), and even earned a Nobel Prize in Economics in 2002, discussing the predictability of heuristic bias. Kahneman's work was not conceived with healthcare in mind as the primary adopter; his theory, however, works convincingly well in healthcare, where if we see something that requires immediate action (a life-threatening problem), or sufficiently simple to make a spot diagnosis (a deformed limb post trauma), little reasoning is required to inform the management plan. Alternatively, if the presenting complaint has an unclear narrative, or does not fit any particular pattern, we ought to switch to System 2 in an attempt to figure out what might be occurring.

Croskerry (2009), initially devised a visual model of universal reasoning in healthcare that applies the two systems of dual process theory and how doctors can reach a diagnostic conclusion. Through the author's (SR) current research and thesis on decision-making, it is emerging that paramedics also use a similar dual process of intuition-analytic-intuition to derive an appropriate outcome (see Figure 3.4 as a developing example).

There are, however, several issues with dual process theory (and consequently the models).

Suppose for instance, we have little to no idea about the condition that is presented before us (as in the urticaria example). Since there is no pattern to recognize and

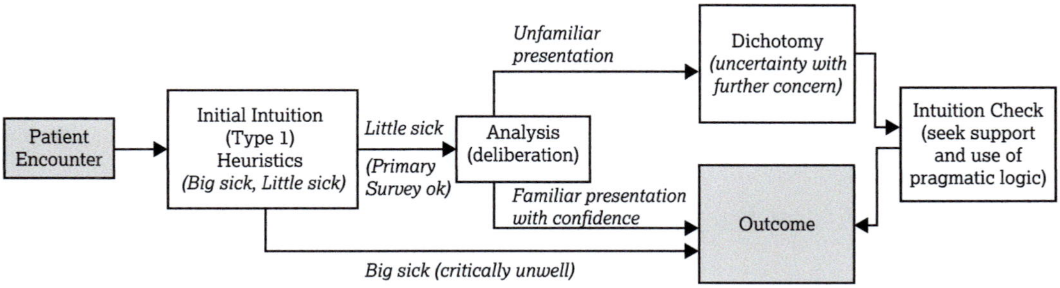

Figure 3.4 Example model of paramedic dual-process reasoning.
Source: Robinson, unpublished thesis

no prior knowledge to draw further information, we are left to think abductively or share the decision with someone who may know. Moreover, in prehospital paramedic practice we may then struggle to reflect and build on knowledge and experience, as there is unlikely to be a follow up as to what the condition might have been. Remember, though, that golden rule #4 advocates for a sensible approach in these situations; it is impossible to know everything and, as paramedics, there is a stronger argument for ruling out significant conditions and formulating an appropriate management plan than there is for demonstrating diagnostic prowess.

Another issue with dual process when applied to healthcare is the linearity of the theory. Is it not possible to be logical without being intuitive? If this were the case, then System 2 would be able to initiate itself and therefore the process isn't particularly 'dual'. When starting any game, such as chess, there may be a logical plan in place prior to any pattern formation. The same applies to paramedics responding to an incident. For example, the ambulance dispatch screen may state 'collapsed male not breathing'; a good paramedic will start considering the range of possibilities and drawing up a plan – System 2. Of course, upon arrival the dispatch rationale may be completely different from the presenting complaint, and thus System 2 reverts to System 1. Or the plan matches the presentation and therefore System 2 can continue. Critical care paramedics, in particular, may be adopting such an approach simply because they know what they are going to (although this needs to be evidenced further).

Considering these points, De Neys (2012, 2014) proposed the concept of **logical intuition**, which is best described as anything that innately conflicts with heuristics. Or, in other words, examples of common sense, prior knowledge of principles, or being autonomously aware of biases and pitfalls. Some examples include Frankenstein being a monster (he was the scientist that created the monster), being 'blind as a bat' (bats can see), or the odds that 23 people in a room share a birthday is 253:1 (it's actually 50:50); you won't be as easily fooled the next time any of these facts next make an appearance, and if you already knew the correct answers, then System 2 wasn't required to think about recalling them (unless you had forgotten them!). This is an example of logical intuition. The previous example on urticaria illustrates logical intuition in practice, as there was no particular pattern that matched to anything obvious, such as an allergic reaction. Yet, if you previously knew urticaria was associated with other conditions, this shouldn't have taken much further thought. Other instances include inaccurate narratives, such as with people suffering from dementia or having to make the snap decision as to whether the individual in front of you is experiencing an expected end of life event.

Naturalistic Decision Making

In contrast to dual process theory, which can sometimes be difficult to apply to the complexities of the real world of healthcare, with its time pressures and dynamic relationships and experiences between clinicians and patients, is 'naturalistic decision theory'. This was originally introduced in 1989 by a team of researchers including Klein and Orasanu, who explored decision making in natural environments, such as how Fire Ground Commanders used heuristics as a means to form mental models that rapidly form a singular decision – a preferred course of action (Klein et al., 1993). This is thought to be particularly useful when under pressure.

The mental models, which can be thought of as scripts, are patterns and processes that are familiar and can be followed. This is slightly different from heuristics because it naturally follows a pre-existing action plan that has become a form of '**tacit knowledge**', which is not dissimilar to De Neys's concept of logical intuition. It is important to note here that action plans are processes that can either be learned formally, such as taught in university paramedic science programmes (arguably generic processes), or learned through experience (unique and individualized scripts). In paramedic practice this form of scripting can be observed during a cardiac arrest:

1. Primary survey.
2. Confirm cardiac arrest – request additional resources.
3. Commence basic life support, attach defibrillation pads, chest compressions, 360 access, prepare airway.
4. Prepare advanced life support.
5. Initiate advanced life support.

It simply wouldn't feel natural to jump in at step 3 or 4 without having progressed through 1 and 2. However, if we consider that the cardiac arrest may actually be an end of life event, limited in additional resources, or consisting of a difficult extrication, then the script must naturally deviate, resulting in a new mental model. Anderson et al.'s study (2021) exploring resuscitation decisions of ambulance personnel in New Zealand demonstrated just that, concluding that decisions to commence or cease resuscitation efforts were naturally contingent on many real-world factors, such as knowledge, experience, motivation, status of the patient and control of the scene.

Little is known, though, about how applicable the model is to low-acuity situations or scenarios that require a multi-disciplinary approach. Additionally, it is not obvious whether naturalistic decision making allows for critical reflection – to change one's mind or acknowledge that an error has been made and calibrate accordingly. Whereas certain situations in paramedic practice need a specific action plan, many do not, and thus naturalistic decision making as a theory lacks versatility in comparison to dual process theory.

The Cognitive Continuum

Both dual process theory and naturalistic decision making have similar elements, incorporating heuristics and intuitions, the former with analytical thinking and the latter attempting to acknowledge the intricacies of the real world. Remember that both theories try to explain how decisions are made, and there is yet to be a theory that either combines the two or completely explains human cognition.

Paramedics, however, are not destined to adhere to one particular theory or style of reasoning, and can learn to become better decision makers. It is considered that the theories and concepts discussed in this chapter can be placed on a continuum, enabling the clinician to adopt a decision-making style that is appropriate for the demands and complexities of the situation. This is known as the **cognitive continuum**. We will go into more detail about this model in the following chapter after further discussion surrounding the dark side of decision making – **error** – because even well-reasoned decisions can go wrong.

Patient Safety: Error, Blame and Just Culture

Essential Recommended Reading

There is an ever-growing drive within healthcare to understand and apply human factors (HF) and **ergonomics** – how we improve the way humans interact with tasks and environments. You should consider reading *Human Factors in Paramedic Practice* (Rutherford, 2020) as an accompaniment to the topic of decision making, as it provides valuable insights for decision-makers working in complex healthcare systems.

This edition of the book continues to support and reflect the principles of applied human factors for paramedics in practice. The origins of HF in healthcare in the UK are in many ways attributable to Martin Bromiley, whose experiences continue to resonate and are captured in the short film called 'Just a Routine Operation'. It is hoped that the content of the film will give you greater insight into the work done to prevent errors in healthcare, make you strive for greater understanding of what factors create error, and consider more the importance of humility when things go wrong. You can find the film by typing this link into your browser (https://www.youtube.com/watch?v=JzlvgtPlof4) or by searching in Google for 'Just a Routine Operation'. Further resources are also available from the Clinical Human Factors Group, a charity set up by Martin Bromiley (https://chfg.org/).

Healthcare is not without risk for any party involved: patient, caregiver, family, public or the system itself. It has been suggested that, despite striving to prevent harm, adverse events arising from healthcare are inevitable, and it has been argued that the notion of 'never events' is unattainable (HSSIB, 2021c). While that may be challenged on both sides, and forms an important consideration regarding safety and reliability in healthcare, the position remains that patients and staff may come to harm, both physically and psychologically, as a result of interacting with healthcare. This should not infer any reduction in our collective focus on providing safe and effective care, rather that the focus should shift towards system design to mitigate risks and, where humans are being relied upon, that tasks and processes are optimally developed.

For the decision maker, understanding the associated hazards and consequences of dealing with the socio-technical endeavour of providing healthcare, particularly high-acuity, complex undifferentiated care, will help minimize risk. Safety relies upon the presence of reliable system components (Weick and Sutcliffe, 2015) and therefore the good decision maker may be considered as being a vital component in a safe system. An additional consideration in healthcare must therefore be to be mindful of the system you work in, the reliability of its components, and its overall safety.

> *If the system lets you make the error, it is badly designed. And if the system induces you to make the error, then it is really badly designed.*
>
> (Norman, 2013)

Other safety critical industries have, over recent decades, wrestled with the realities of the likelihood of failures that can lead to harm. The emergence of greater understanding of the nature of failure has to some degree informed differing approaches to prevention or acceptance within systems, and how risks are tolerated or removed. There are two broad approaches that have described the way organizations approach the risks associated with the service they provide, be it in manufacturing, banking or healthcare, and regardless of the type of jeopardy, such as injury/death, interruption in trading or financial failures. These two approaches are known as 'normal accident theory' – accepting that bad things will happen and learning from those events – and 'high reliability organizing' – seeking to understand what could go wrong before things do – based around five key principles, which coalesce into a safety system.

- **Preoccupation with failure** – continually studying and monitoring the system for integrity and failure.
- **Reluctance to simplify** – accepting that systems are complex and designing ways to manage this.
- **Sensitivity to the operation** – awareness of the stressors and load on a system that will affect quality and safety, rather than simply performance.
- **Commitment to resilience** – creating systems designed to maintain their function across a predicted range.

- **Deference to expertise** – listening to people nearest the problem and/or reaching out to those who know the most (as opposed to those paid the most).

(Weick & Sutcliffe, 2015)

These are important considerations for decision makers delivering care, as normal accident theory makes allowance for things going wrong and actually relies on those events as a basis for new learning. This approach necessitates operators sharing their experiences and facing the fear of (or being the actual victim of) adverse consequences professionally.

System Safety and Reliability

High-reliability organizing states that adverse events are not inevitable and that by focusing on the reliability of system components, the overall enterprise can be safe. This approach is reflected in the difference between Safety 1 and Safety 2 (Hollnagel, Wears and Braithwaite, 2015)[1] and can help clinicians in practice contextualize their role in what is commonly a closely coupled system (that is to say, a system where things happen quickly with limited opportunity to stop to think). Safety 1 requires an event upon which an investigation takes place in order to elicit learning, whereas Safety 2 seeks to understand systems without an event to predict and prevent failures.

Examples of processes that are closely coupled include rocket launches and rollercoaster rides: once commenced, they are very hard to stop. In healthcare, we should challenge ourselves to understand which of our processes are necessarily coupled (for instance, surgical procedures or resuscitation), which operate in a cascade of actions ('hierarchical tasks') and have close interdependencies, and which are loosely coupled. Process coupling also requires an understanding of the level of management the endeavour needs. Plate-spinning is a closely coupled and intensively managed endeavour, as the plates will stop spinning if the sticks are not attended to frequently. For paramedics, we sometimes need to consider whether the patient's journey can be decoupled in order to be optimized. For example, taking a patient to the emergency department at midnight versus not transporting and suggesting an alternative care plan for the following morning. The pressure to complete an episode of care within a culture of perceived or actual pressure (such as on-scene times for paramedics in an ambulance setting, or the movement of patients through a fast track area of a hospital) may be the result of a poorly designed system that fails to appreciate its own moving parts.

As clinicians we have personal accountability for the decisions we make and the actions we take; however, being aware of the systems in which we work and striving to enhance their design and reliability will become an increasing priority for healthcare professionals as a method ensuring their intrinsic fallibilities are

[1] **N.B.** Take care not to confuse Safety 1 and Safety 2 with System-1 and System-2 thinking!

considered along with the tools of the trade, the physical environment and the culture of the organization.

The Nature of Errors, Mistakes and Violations

> *While a particular practice or omission may be the immediate cause of an incident, closer analysis usually reveals a series of events and departures from safe practice, each influenced by the working environment and the wider organisational context.*
>
> (Vincent and Taylor-Adams, 2001)

If we agree that human beings are fallible and are simply one of numerous components within a complex system, we should therefore analyse the failure modes and their effects that befall humans in order for us to learn and improve and understand failure more broadly. Safety science provides analytical models that help us to understand how systems work (and fail). For example, 'SEIPS' (systems engineering initiative in patient safety) or 'FMEA' (Failure Mode Effects Analysis) are used to understand the components of a work system, how they form processes and lead to outcomes, along with the influence of adaptation (Holden et al., 2013) within the Donabedian system: structure (work systems), processes and outcomes (Donabedian, 2005). While centrally positioned within the work system, the *person* (worker) is interconnected with the other factors, such as the *environment* and *tools and technology* (see Figure 3.5). When we consider errors in healthcare practice – a drug error, for example – if we apply blame, we risk missing the factors that may have been designed into the work system, and which have existed latently until an event occurs. This in turn prevents improvement and does not address the safety risk, not to mention the psychological risk to the clinician.

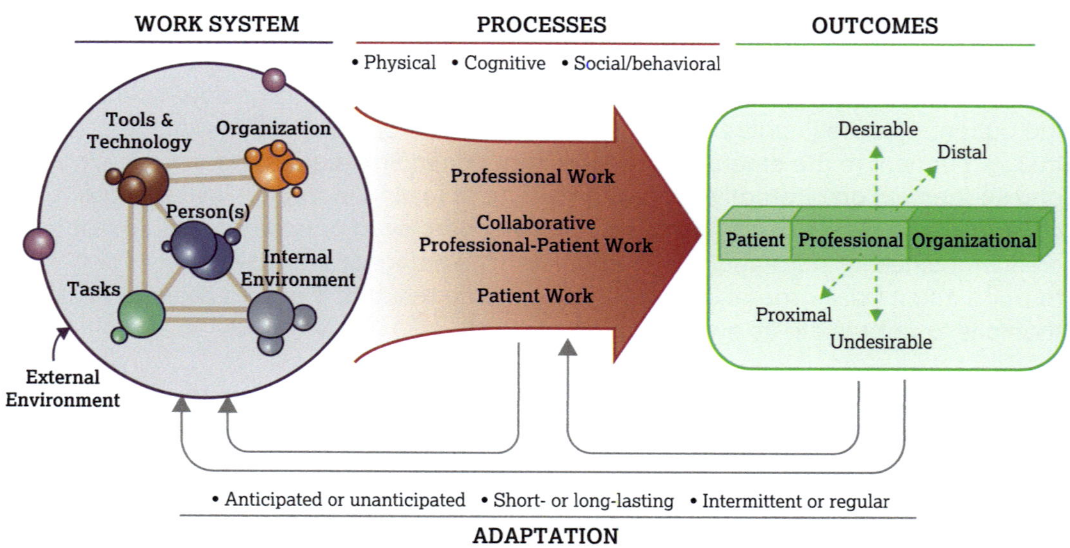

Figure 3.5 SEIPS 2.0 (System Engineering Initiative in Patient Safety).
Source: Holden et al., 2013.

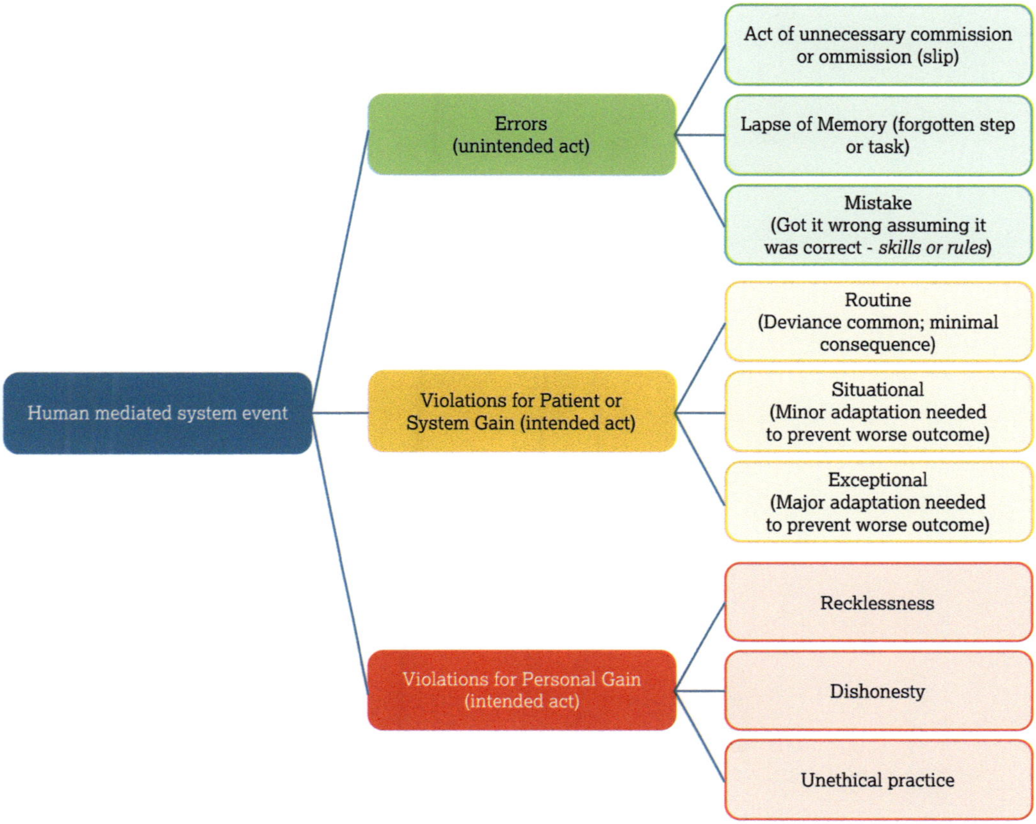

Figure 3.6 What is a mistake? What is an error? Words have meanings.

The detection of incidents or events, if not identified prior to an event using Safety 2 principles (design it out before it happens), usually requires a human interaction (act of commission or omission), generally in the form of an 'error' as a catch-all term. However, in the context of understanding human performance as well as psychological wellbeing, it is helpful to classify issues correctly to better understand how they arise and how they can be prevented (see Figure 3.6). For example, mistakes may be due to lapses or gaps in knowledge, errors may be skill based, and violations may or may not be attitudinal in origin. In the broader context of error prevention and management, the conditions in which the human is working must be considered centrally as a causative factor, rather than the classification of the issue in isolation.

In context, these could be exemplified in the following ways (and see Figure 3.7):

- **Error** – The paramedic gave 1 mg of adrenaline 1:1000. They drew up the entire volume of the vial but forgot to stop the administration at 500 mcg – *Skill-based error.*
- **Violation** – The paramedic did not record a blood glucose reading as they stated that the patient, who had twisted their ankle, was not diabetic. This is contrary to organizational policy – *Attitudinal error.*

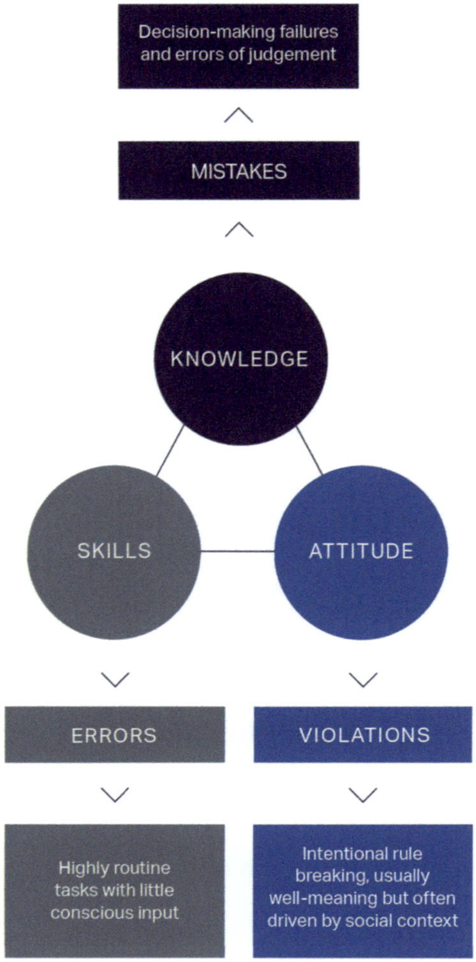

Figure 3.7 Originally the FAiR® system graphic, is reproduced with kind permission of Baines Simmons.

Source: Baines Simmons Ltd, 2019

- **Mistake** – The paramedic felt that the abdominal pain was due to the patient's ongoing gastrointestinal problems. They did not know that the patient's symptoms could indicate a potential new, additional, acute abdominal disorder – *Knowledge-based error.*

Before moving on, it is important to recognize that healthcare workers do not want to cause harm. While history sadly tells us that there are extremely rare exceptions, such as Harold Shipman and Beverley Allitt, the harm these people cause is premeditated and on a scale that most of us cannot even start to comprehend. Healthcare staff go to work to do a good job to the best of their ability and are also impacted negatively as a result of accidents and errors. The impact on healthcare workers involved in harm events is becoming better understood and is referred to as 'second victim phenomenon' (the patient being the first victim) (Dekker, 2013).

Importantly, the knowledge, skill, dedication and vigilance of healthcare workers provide an incredible level of error and harm prevention and mitigation, despite the poorly designed conditions seen commonly in healthcare settings.

The anguish caused to healthcare workers involved in harm events demonstrates tangibly that caregivers do not set out to harm patients. There are, however, times when this is not the case and harm is caused due to violations arising from an intention to make personal gain (as opposed to gain for the patient's or organization's benefit). There are also occasions where errors arise from egregious or wilful negligence (underpinning the importance of CPD), or even cases where acts are intended to harm patients or sabotage an organization. Part of professional practice for paramedics as decision makers is to understand the ethical and legal basis for practice and to strive to operate within the expectations of that designation, as laid out by the provincial legislation and/or regulations, standards and in key publications such as *Law and Ethics for Paramedics: An Essential Guide* (Eaton, 2024).

Error and blame must therefore be understood and contextualized to ensure that healthcare professionals can practice with confidence and with cognitive freedom, unburdened by anxiety and the fear of punitive action arising from the unintended consequences of action undertaken in good faith, and within a complex socio-technical system that may not be well designed or safe.

Blame and Moving Towards a Just Culture

Why do we apportion blame to others or ourselves, and what is blame?

> *. . . to say or think that someone did something wrong or is responsible for something bad happening.*
>
> (Cambridge Dictionary)

Blame is, in simple terms, human nature, and is perhaps used as a strategy to seek resolution and to move on or to exact a form of justice. The problem with blame is that it is by its very nature applied retrospectively, following a pathway of detection, investigation and attribution (at the expense of learning), and is assessed using expected norms and in the absence of the situational context. That is to say that the attribution is made in the cold light of day, based on the presumption of optimal conditions, and with evidence used subjectively and influenced by hindsight. It is far too easy to say 'you shouldn't have done that', and resolve the episode without looking beyond the detection event. Healthcare incident investigations are modernizing and improving but have historically relied upon 'root cause analysis', which, in healthcare applications and with the exclusion of associated analytical techniques, assumes that untoward events are linear and rely on the holes in the Swiss cheese lining up (James Reason). Modern methods of understanding incidents, such as those used by the Air Accident Investigation Branch (AAIB, 2021), and which were subsequently adopted by the Healthcare Safety Investigation Branch (HSIB, 2021a), use the emergence or 'reference event' as the starting point of an investigation. By understanding the safety risk using a range of analytical methodologies, such as SEIPS (which was discussed earlier), FRAM, STAMP, AcciMap and Accident Route Matrix, the complex interconnecting constellation of factors are elicited and presented in a way that allows systemic recommendations to be made, rather than blaming an individual and/or asking the human beings to be more vigilant.

As healthcare moves towards a truly embedded 'just culture', which focuses on learning and reducing harm for all stakeholders, clinicians such as paramedics, who are on the frontline and making often complex clinical decisions in the heat of battle, will also need to adopt a growth mindset and learn to trust this new cultural dawn.

Where egregious or wilful negligence is not a factor, and personal gain is proven to not be a driver, clinicians must seek to share their experiences in practice with confidence that the act of speaking up does not in itself carry negative consequence. A just culture must include psychological safety for staff and feature mechanisms that protect from moral injury in the same way employers strive to avoid back injuries or needle-stick injuries. This relies on trust between all parties, and clinicians including in their decision-making acumen a conscious decision to share their failures, mistakes and errors. While Safety 1 driven learning (reactive – only investigating and learning after an event) will always remain in healthcare, albeit we hope only residually in the future, we must embrace the reporting culture necessary to drive learning, but also to start speaking up about things that might go wrong but have not yet. The concept of appreciative inquiry, looking for 'weak signals' (CIEHF, 2020), and quality improvement activities must form a greater part of healthcare professionals' job planning and objectives.

Healthcare is risky. Borrowing from a Twitter thread by Ken Catchpole (MUSC, n.d.), which underpins the inevitable nature of harm, it was suggested that unlike machines, which are deterministic and predictable, patients are non-deterministic and unpredictable; the drug error that has no adverse effect on one patient, could kill another.

It is important to remember that a *just culture* must be everyone's lived experience, and we must also embrace a *learning culture*. We cannot select which elements of these we follow, and we cannot turn a blind eye to those weak signals that, if not reported, could prevent improvements to safety. **Cognitive dissonance** can affect how we approach certain aspects of our personal and professional lives. We cannot demand fairness for ourselves but not promote justice for our patients and colleagues. To make our systems of care safer, we must be courageous, report what we see, and be prepared to work on improvements as an intrinsic aspect of practice, which is arguably as tangible as direct patient care.

Activity

Think about a common error or a specific error or mistake you have experienced. Break down the task itself and consider how the process was designed.

- What were the issues?
- Was anyone right or wrong?

- What were the actual problems?
- Whose 'fault' was it (person/system/other)?

Think about the nature of the event and the consequences as you perceived them versus that actual outcome. What would you change, both in terms of the task and process and the subsequent actions that follow such an event?

You can expand your understanding of tools like SEIPS by reading the following paper:

- Web Link: https://www.ncbi.nlm.nih.gov/pmc/articles/PMC3835697/
- Search 'SEIPS 2.0'

Checklists and Structured Communication

The Clinical Human Factors Group (2015) defines a checklist as: '*A job aid designed to concisely summarize the key elements of a task as an aid to memory and ensure correct procedures are followed*'.

It is entirely unrealistic for human beings to retain the volume of information published in the healthcare literature and guidance, and yet we commonly see omissions attributed to 'human error' (such as forgetting something). These can be more specifically assessed as relating to the challenges that humans face in day-to-day life. We must recognize the true nature of human error if we want to embrace a learning culture. The term '**no blame culture**' is commonly used, but 'learning culture' better describes how issues must be kept on the radar rather than being connected with someone or something under the banner of blame.

Were we to replace our human professional workforce with automatons, we wouldn't need to worry about the limitations associated with humans – fatigue, stress, hunger, personal problems, shift working, illness etc. – as machines don't get tired or hungry, they are not moved by emotional experiences, they don't have arguments with their partners or have any stress. They could store all the information they would ever need in an infinitely expandable hard-drive and be able to recall expertly every disease and treatment, regardless how infrequently they presented. The problem with this hypothetical example is, of course, that even if these robots existed (yet), the patient would receive little or no care or compassion – core tenets of healthcare (NHS England, 2014a). So, we tolerate the limitations of humans because the essence of healthcare relies on higher concepts, such as empathy. The next best thing to trying to create a caring robot is to help humans behave in a more robot-like way at times where recall may be affected by extrinsic factors. This is where checklists come in.

Checklists have existed in the airline industry for decades, and every aspect of an aircraft's flight is covered by a checklist: *before-start, after-start, before take-off, after take-off/climb, approach, landing, after-landing, parking* – to name but a few. Each of these checklists serve to remove variations from the process and remove the risk of omission – a very simple principle but one which has not had the same level of adoption in healthcare, except for a few very notable examples, such as the WHO Surgical Checklist (WHO, 2008), which has reduced surgical errors by over 30%. Checklists are most useful where the endeavour has the highest risk (such as the sign-in element of the WHO surgical checklist) and where the environment and team are focused on the task being checked. A report by the Healthcare Safety Investigation Branch (HSIB, 2020) noted that the sign-out phase may be less diligently applied due to competing priorities within the operating team.

One area of paramedic practice that has fully embraced the use of checklists is critical care paramedicine, where high-risk interventions are undertaken using detailed checklists to prepare equipment and identify roles and responsibilities, what drugs are being given and, very importantly, what the contingencies are should things go wrong. The checklist process also introduces more clear and structured communication, setting up the team in such a way that minimizes risks of miscommunication.

Checklists have four main types (static parallel, static sequential with verification, static sequential with verification and confirmation, and dynamic) (Winters et al., 2009), but in essence they all work by providing a prompt that requires a response. Checklists can function with a single person, or a whole team, and the level of variation is informed by the level of certainty required.

It is important to consider checklists as a strong ally, and not something which diminishes your professional status. It is not a requirement of practice to remember everything, and the fact is most people cannot go shopping without forgetting something important unless they write a shopping list. It is unlikely anyone would base their ego and sense of self-worth on the basis of remembering a shopping list, so why would healthcare professionals seek to remember the list of things that need doing – particularly when we consider the hostile and dynamic environments in which we practise. Our patients will not be impressed with our powers of recall were we able to remember everything that needs doing. In contrast, though, if we fail to recall something vital, the negative effect on them may be huge.

Human Fallibility and Biased Thinking – Learn Before You Make Mistakes

We will explore how bias can affect decision making in Chapter 4, and throughout this book, we talk of distractions, fallacies and biases. But what does this actually mean?

Before we move on, please watch the following film (either type 'Monkey Business Illusion' into a search engine or type the link below into your browser) to undertake a quick test of your ability to concentrate and your susceptibility to distractions (Simons, 2010).

- Web Link: https://www.youtube.com/watch?v=IGQmdoK_ZfY
- Search 'Monkey Business Illusion'

Daniel Kahneman's work on the way we as humans think touched on the way external influences and biases can be managed (Kahneman, 2012). Who saw the gorilla in the YouTube clip, but missed the player leaving and the curtain changing colour? To expand on this, and to ensure that these concepts can be recognized and managed when applying a decision-making process, the different influences (such as distraction and bias) that can be identified have been expanded with examples of where they can affect decisions and outcomes.

It is worth bearing in mind that Daniel Kahneman is not a healthcare professional, rather he is a psychologist and economist. Many of his examples relate to decision making in economics, and none relate directly to healthcare. There is a good reason why the word 'clinical' is not used in the context of 'clinical decision making' in this book – as decision making is a human endeavour, and the subject matter which is affected by the decision is domain-agnostic. You can misdiagnose a patient, choose the wrong investment portfolio, or buy the wrong size jumper in the clothes store – all based on the same fallibilities associated with the psychology of decision making. With this in mind, decision-making skills are transferrable across all aspects of your life (a rare thing in healthcare), so enjoy.

The next section will look first at those biases put forward by Kahneman which relate most relevantly to clinical practice, after which examples of other relevant biases and fallacies, are explored with practice examples.

Anchoring

Anchoring is the effect where we tend to allow ourselves to be influenced by numbers that may be irrelevant. While this is most prevalent in consumer psychology – setting a price-point that is acceptable to customers upon which all other prices are set – healthcare has many numbers associated with it, mainly the display of physiological values on monitoring devices, which are contextualized against an anchored normal range.

How often have you looked at a patient who is clearly not unwell, but the pulse oximeter shows a heart rate of 250 BPM and oxygen saturations of 45%? We tend to believe what we see because we anchor a nominal normal for these values, and more usually have a low tolerance for values that appear catastrophic. In this case, a poor signal is almost always the problem and while considering intervention is appropriate, the global picture of the patient leads you to review the quality of the data first.

Consider the 65 kg female involved in a minor collision in their car. 'Normal' blood pressure is 120/80, but this patient's BP is 85/55 – is this abnormal? Is the patient compensating? When you consider the wider picture, and on speaking to the patient (who you are trying to wrestle onto to the trolley in order to raise her legs in the air) she reports that this is her normal blood pressure. If this scenario involved a 200 kg male, the anchoring would be more useful. In this case, though, it's a heuristic bias.

Availability

We tend to err towards that which is available mentally or practically. **Ideation** can be linked to the bias of availability and can have strange logical outcomes. For example, does working in an ambulance increase the chances of deciding to take a patient to hospital compared to when working on a response car? Does the presence of the availability of transport make the decision easier as it's more available? Clearly, the decision to convey must be based on the patient's needs, and not extrinsic factors.

Also, availability is linked to the consequence of a decision and the perception of its outcome where the thought is close at hand. For example, imagine a hypothetical scenario where you are working at an ambulance station where a colleague was recently the subject of an investigation following a complaint about discharging a patient from scene. While the investigation demonstrated no case to answer, the anxiety relating to being investigated may have increased the number of patients taken to hospital in the period following the investigation, compared to the neighbouring station in the same city. The most available thought was related to consequence, and this, in turn, affected decisions for patients despite the actual or statistical chance of facing disciplinary action from a complaint (particularly if you make good decisions).

Conjunction Bias

'Conjunction' is simply where events happen at the same time, and where it occurs as a bias it explains where the connection of events can lead to a connection of cause – sometimes incorrectly.

Poorly made intuitive judgements can be highly unethical, and seriously compromise clinical practice, where the **conjunction bias** is present. For example, is it more likely that the incident you are responding to will be perceived negatively if the patient with 'chest pain' is a homeless person than if the patient is living in a detached house in suburbia? This judgement can play out, and the homeless person's needs may not match the initial call. But likewise, the call to the middle-class home may also yield a judgement that it would have been better to see a pharmacist or go to the GP. The important consideration is that if you *must* judge the appropriateness of a 911 call, you should only do it at the end of the incident! Providing subjective information as a series of attributes in a conjoined way, and in an unweighted way, creates a picture that may belie the actual need. The way in which patients enter urgent and emergency care systems makes conjunction more likely, as the information is often truncated and lacks context.

The conjunction bias was discovered through an experiment that Kahneman carried out, called 'The Linda Problem', which provided some very scant information about a made-up subject. Those taking part in the experiment were asked to consider the most likely answer. The research subjects were told that Linda is 'young, single, outspoken, and very bright, who, as a student, was deeply concerned with discrimination and social justice' (Kahneman and Tversky, 1983), and were then asked to decide if Linda was a 'bank teller' or a 'feminist bank teller'. The question omits the qualifying statements needed to avoid making a decision which in terms of probability is less likely, and the outcome showed the majority of the subject's assumed Linda was a feminist. In terms of probability, the chances of Linda being a bank teller are significantly higher than her being a feminist bank teller, and the information provided gives no definite suggestion of feminism. The conjunction of the information led to the unconscious bias.

The issue relates to what is implied rather than what is correct, avoiding the instinctive answer, and this requires parking all assumptions and social taboos. When making decisions in practice, consider carefully the information you are provided with compared to the information you may seek to elicit. The latter is easier to qualify and can help avoid the conjunction bias.

Optimism and Loss Aversion

In the next chapter, we look at how we approach what we know and what we may not know (**known knowns**, **known unknowns** etc.) and this demonstrates how much we tend towards optimism and overconfidence. In practice, clinicians may be inclined towards optimism or pessimism due to their previous experience of a particular disease or patient outcome, and if pessimism develops it may impede good decision making due to the phenomenon of '**loss aversion**'. For instance, this may mean that it is preferred to get every patient with a pulse to hospital regardless of the prognosis rather than 'call it' on scene, as this removes the perceived loss, or guards against unrealistic expectations of the outcome. It could be argued that, in paramedic practice, the balance between optimism and pessimism occurs on a patient-by-patient basis; for example, the patient whose injuries are clearly incompatible with life but for whom everything is done to demonstrate absolute futility by evidencing no response to all available interventions, is approached with determination, but ultimately pessimism. Conversely, the patient you hand over at hospital, for whom the long-term outcome is unclear, is left with a feeling of optimism. Either way, the aversion to loss in the healthcare setting is not healthy for the clinician, and needs to be understood and recognized so that perhaps all patients can be approached optimistically and also realistically (Kahneman, 2012).

There are dozens of biases and fallacies that have been identified in human psychology, many of which are relevant to healthcare decision making. The 2013 book by Rolf Dobelli, referenced earlier in this chapter, presents a list of 100 biases and fallacies. Dobelli collates these into a series of real-world examples which support the title *The Art of Thinking Clearly*. Many of these have direct links to the challenges related to decision making in paramedic practice and healthcare in general. They are listed below with practice examples relevant to patient care.

Other Relevant Biases and Fallacies

Confirmation Bias

The writer Aldous Huxley said that facts do not cease to exist if they are simply ignored, and confirmation bias is where information is omitted or altered to fit a more convenient answer. This is at the heart of good decision making and is the basis for ensuring good hypotheses are created and tested, and that the unknown unknowns are considered. This bias is always at the top of the list as it requires key professional attributes, such as insight and humility, in order to prevent problems.

The patient who 'fits' nicely into a diagnosis by omitting the confounding factors is at risk of their clinician being subject to confirmation bias. For example, the 39-year-old male with no family history of cardiovascular disease, and who has a three-day history of fever and productive cough, must be suffering chest pain due to his chest infection. He has been coughing a lot and is *too young to be having a heart attack* (a dangerous assumption with cardiac sounding chest pain).

WRONG – he is *ALSO* having a **myocardial infarction** and will be dead within the next three hours.

Authority Bias

The airline industry, as mentioned at the start of the chapter, has learned much about **authority bias** in its development of CRM (cockpit resource management), which has further developed in wider settings to 'crew resource management'. The basic premise of CRM is that the most senior person isn't always correct, and the hierarchies can conspire to cause sometimes catastrophic outcomes, as we saw in the example involving Martin Bromiley's wife.

One of the key examples of authority bias was the Tenerife air disaster on 27th March 1977. This demonstrated the issue of the relationship between levels of authority and status (captain versus first officer) regarding who was wrong, and the inability of the junior pilot whose belief was correct (Aviation Safety Network, n.d.).

Luckily for paramedics, our practice settings are more and more in tune with CRM. The risk of authority bias still exists, and we must be prepared to speak up. For example, the very new ED staff physician who wishes to proceed with a procedural sedation after the department paramedic has identified this patient as high risk can be approached in a polite and professional way and will be receptive to the challenge. This will mean the patient gets the best care.

Outcome/Hindsight Bias

It is important to judge each decision on the process used rather than the outcome. This links closely to the need to be very cautious if basing your practice entirely upon experience and intuition as the diagnoses, treatment choices and outcomes may merely be a long string of lucky guesses!

A good decision may lead to the wrong answer, and a bad decision can lead to the correct answer. Regardless of the outcome, however, a poorly made decision is always the wrong answer. In other words, judge the outcome on how you arrived at the answer rather than the answer itself. Using a decision-making process makes practice as safe as possible and allows the clinician to focus on the patient's episode of care, rather than just whether the outcome is optimized.

Overconfidence Bias

We all like to think we get things right most of the time, but humans are intrinsically prone to overestimating their ability, and focus on positive experiences when assessing competency.

In clinical care, forecasting what is wrong with the patient based on the confidence of the clinician is a potentially dangerous way to make complex decisions. **Experiential** and entirely intuitive decision making is covered in subsequent chapters, and the associated concepts that exist alongside overconfidence must be understood by clinicians in order to promote good care for patients. Professional insight and humility are opportunities to promote healthy levels of confidence in practice.

It is possible that an unbroken run of absence of failure can lead to overconfidence in subsequent encounters; feeding a false sense of security built up over time. This can also link to the authority-biased behaviours where the overconfident clinician demonstrates poor leadership due to overconfidence in their ability and an unwillingness to be challenged.

Try this quick exercise. How many diseases could you name that are linked to a chief complaint of abdominal pain? Next, estimate the diagnostic certainty you have when assessing patients with abdominal pain. The literature suggests that diagnoses associated with abdominal pain are wrong 50% of the time, and the list of conditions is upwards of 50. If you named half the conditions, and accept the published diagnostic accuracy, there is little grounds for overconfidence!

Base-rate Neglect

This bias is linked to 'The Linda Problem' (Tversky and Kahneman, 1982) and highlights the issue with failing to appreciate the underlying statistical probabilities of the decisions you make. Consider the following variation on the Linda Problem.

Chuck is white, lives in Los Angeles and has committed two murders. Is Chuck most likely to be (A) a member of a Hells Angels motorcycle chapter, or (B) a corporate lawyer?

There are 1.2 million lawyers in the USA, and, according to the US Justice Department, only 2,500 Hells Angels worldwide. So, while it seems most plausible that Chuck is a Hells Angels member, it is statistically more likely that he is a lawyer. The intuitive leap to assuming he is a Hells Angel is an example of **base-rate neglect**.

While good decision making should always be aware that rare things happen (rarely), the most likely outcome is most likely. In healthcare, the challenge is to prove that Chuck ISN'T a member of the Hells Angels, rather than proving he is lawyer. Using abdominal pain again as an example, a 14-year-old male with **right iliac fossa** tenderness is most likely to have appendicitis but could also have an **ischaemic bowel** or a **hernia**. The base rate instance of appendicitis is far greater than the other two differential diagnoses, both of which must be excluded, along with other significant potential pathologies.

False Causality Bias

A very obvious example of **false causality** is how low blood glucose can mimic very closely stroke symptoms. Consider this real-world example from an Ambulance Technician, working alongside a paramedic colleague:

Case Study: False Causality Bias

We were shown to a patient's bedroom and after a couple of minutes became suspicious about how she was presenting. On doing some simple observations, including blood glucose testing, we found her to be profoundly hypoglycaemic, and reversed this with glucagon (a medicine that mobilizes stores of glucose from the liver). As she began to wake, I was tasked by the paramedic to find some oral carbohydrates, and so went down to ask the family if they had any digestive biscuits. They seemed a little surprised that the ambulance crew were peckish enough to ask for biscuits, and I did fail to provide the full update at that stage.

Fifteen minutes later, we walked the patient down the stairs into the living room to gasps of shock from the family. We explained what happened and placed a call to the GP to say what we had done, and would he still like us to take her to hospital, or would he like to return to make a further assessment. He chose to send her in.

This case highlights the risk of leaping to an obvious conclusion based on false causality. The signs and symptoms suggested stroke, but this was not the correct diagnosis. Stroke, along with hypoglycaemia, should have been a hypothesis (differential diagnosis) at this stage.

Action Bias

'Quick, do something!' Paramedics often hear this when they arrive at an incident, and it can jolt us into 'action bias' – doing something rather than nothing to avoid appearing ineffective. Many actions are very useful to buy time (such as taking a pulse, for instance), but where a decision is made rashly, using only intuition rather than consideration, it may be harmful. Clearly, there are times when immediate action is the only sensible course of action, such as starting CPR where a patient is pulseless, but where these actions can cause further problems, taking time to consider next steps is vital. The tendency towards action bias is often considered in human factors, and the mantra '10 seconds for 10 minutes' is often used to describe how not acting and spending a few seconds sense checking can save so much more time if the alternative is spending 10 minutes undoing the wrong thing.

In high pressure situations, it takes strong leadership to avoid action bias, and the 10 seconds you spend thinking can feel like a lifetime but is usually a stitch in time!

Omission Bias

Omission bias may be seen at the opposite of action bias, but it is a little more involved than that. Omission bias is best described by the term often heard in healthcare settings – 'if in doubt, don't'. Arguably, this term is outmoded and may be hard to defend.

Consider this scenario: an American paramedic moves to the UK and joins his local ambulance service. It is the early 1990s and he is surprised how few interventions UK paramedics can do compared to the US. A few weeks into his time in the UK he is called to a patient choking in a restaurant. Basic manoeuvres are unsuccessful, and so begins to consider undertaking a surgical airway, but is reminded that in the UK this is outside his remit. The patient finally goes into cardiac arrest, secondary to the airway occlusion. The fear of consequence leads the paramedic not to act and he continues with basic techniques and conveying the patient to the nearest emergency department, where a junior doctor carries out an emergency tracheostomy. Sadly, the patient is well beyond help. The hospital complains to the ambulance service asking why someone who is trained was not able to intervene. The ambulance service defends the actions of the paramedic. The coroner cannot provide any comfort to the family in the inquest as the system at the time was biased towards omission.

There were cases in this period where paramedics acted outside their scope of practice (action bias) with variable outcomes depending on the effect on the patient.

Morally it appears hard to justify, and there is no easy answer. Imagine it in these terms: what is the difference between you pushing someone off a cliff and failing to prevent someone falling off a cliff? The outcome is the same – the person dies in the fall – and the influence you have is only different by the physical contact. Consider the difference of patient outcomes in the context of not acting in a dynamic environment, and the potential end result. Not acting may not be any better than acting. A moral and practical dilemma!

Averages Bias

Averages are very useful in retrospect or at the end of a defined period, such as a season's batting average in cricket, average lap times in motorsport, and response times in ambulance services. The problem with averages is that they take time to settle and can be influenced by large, small, or aberrant data.

Many paramedics lament their poor **ROSC** (return of spontaneous circulation) rates compared to colleagues, or their conveyance rates for all their patients – all in short periods of time. Specialist paramedics in urgent care roles may spend all shift dealing with chest pains and serious trauma, sending all their patients to hospital and achieving a 100% conveyance rate that day. Over the course of a year, that one day will be lost very quickly in the averages, and the successful resuscitations will fluctuate for so many reasons, such as **aetiologies**, demography and geography, to the point where the overall organizational results are unaffected, and all patients receive gold standard care.

The risk of averages is the desire to force them – such as taking more risk with patients discharged from scene in order to reverse a climbing conveyance rate or ignoring advanced directives and resuscitating patients who are not for resuscitation. Imagine a bus carrying 50 people, each earning on average $50,000 dollars per year, is then boarded by Mark Zuckerberg, the founder of Facebook and owner of the Meta empire. At this point, the average earnings on that bus becomes upward of $950m. None of the other passengers feel any richer though. The average is so skewed by the spike that it is rendered useless. On a worldwide level, the influence of Zuckerberg's wealth increases the average by only a few dollars, and yet his personal wealth is unchanged.

Trying to achieve an average is not always helpful, and many quality improvement systems use statistical process control to give upper and lower control limits based on standard deviations from the mean to give a truer and more meaningful display of performance data, as well as provide the opportunity to assess data points that fall outside the upper and lower controls.

Conclusion

This chapter has looked at the cognitive fogs and biases we all suffer as human beings and this leads into the next chapter, where decision-making theories and concepts are pulled together into strategies. Making choices and decisions is, for the most part, an unconscious process. We do not spend large amounts of time choosing what to wear each day, nor are we particularly aware of when we switch on the car headlamps – we simply reach an intuitive judgement based on the weather or reach a threshold at which point we think the lights should go on. These day-to-day decisions are limited in their consequence (we might spend the day feeling cold or get flashed by another motorist to warn us our lights aren't on). Many other decisions are more significant and are blighted by the way we interpret the perceived outcome, and this leads to highly illogical but totally understandable behaviours.

The reference materials that have been cited in this chapter are well worth reading in more depth. The least academic, but most entertaining, book is *The Art of Thinking Clearly* by Rolf Dobelli, and it seems fitting to leave this chapter with a conundrum based on Dobelli's chapter called 'Would you wear Hitler's sweater?', which typifies the human condition using the example of contagion bias.

> *You go into a charity shop and find an old sweater in excellent condition in your size. It is clearly very old indeed, and with antique clothing in demand you think this would make an excellent purchase. You go to the checkout and*

the shopkeeper gives you a very important piece of history about the previous owner of the sweater – it belonged to Adolf Hitler/Jimmy Savile/Ian Brady/ Peter Sutcliffe (delete as appropriate). So, would you wear it? No one will know who it belonged to. It's a bargain, it fits, and it's in excellent condition, so why not? Some decisions will always be fogged by biases and these distractions cannot always be avoided. Who would want to walk around in Hitler's cast-offs, regardless of how illogical it would seem, and yet the emotional response it creates means that the illogical decision is probably the one the majority would go with?

(Based on Dobelli, 2014, pp. 166–168)

So, the decision itself may not be the most important aspect of the episode but navigating your way to the decision certainly is. Thinking back to Chapter 2, can you find your way back to the point where you took each fork in the road? The next chapter opens up a more cyclical and less linear approach, and will start you on a journey to a decision-making acumen.

Reflective Exercises

1. Consider the system you practise in and pick a process that frustrates you. Describe the issues and think about what you would do differently. Challenge yourself to speak up and be part of quality improvement activity, and become part of the design and development of your work.
2. Pick a bias from the list earlier in the chapter and consider a time where you fell victim to the bias you have chosen. This can be in your personal life or professional life. Remember that consumer psychology relies on these biases, so you may want to consider a scenario outside healthcare, perhaps when you made a purchase.
3. Reflect on your autonomy, and your understanding of the term in the context of your professional practice. Consider the human factors relating to team behaviours and safety culture, and how these link to the outcomes for patients.

Chapter 4

Inclusive Decision Making

Sean Teed, Robert Bonspiel, Bo Escritt, Agatha Nortley-Meshe, and Alison Walker

Chapter Objectives

This chapter will cover:

- The importance of equality, diversity and inclusion in the context of diagnosis and decision making
- Health and wellness: a new guiding principle?
- Positionality and the interpretation of life experiences
- What bias is and how it can impact our decision making
- How paramedics can consider and mitigate against bias within their role
- Communication skills, including both verbal communication and body language
- Culture and ethnicity: the impact on disease manifestations and effect on health outcomes.

Why Should We Be Aware of Equality, Diversity and Inclusion?

Paramedics regularly need to make clinical decisions at speed in order to provide the most appropriate medication and best quality care to their patients. Decisions are often made under stressful circumstances and can also be complex, as well as time critical on some occasions. The decisions that paramedics make about treatment can have a serious effect on a patient's life, clinical outcomes, patient safety, health and wellbeing. Therefore, how paramedics come to their judgements and decisions, and what these decisions are based upon, are of paramount importance.

Health and Wellness: A New Guiding Principle?

Health and wellbeing are topics that are taught in many paramedic education programs, or are they? Does health and wellbeing mean the same thing to me as it does to you? Have you ever wondered why so many family members are present in certain calls to the community? Have you sincerely reflected on the *patient* and *family's* idea of wellness?

To answer these questions, it is important to be open to reflecting on two things: positionality and health and wellness through the eyes of others. We will cover to positionality shortly in this chapter, but first we will consider this idea of considering health and wellness through the eyes of others, and specifically the concept of Two-Eyed Seeing.

A personal acknowledgement was introduced at the front of this book, and this acknowledgement penned out the positionality of an individual that included a suggestion to reflect on the 2012 Calls to Action (Truth and Reconciliation Commission of Canada, 2012). Mi' Kmaw Elder Albert Marshall coined the phrase Etuaptmumk/Two-Eyed Seeing. According to Cape Breton University's Institute for Integrative Science and Health, Etuaptmumk/Two-Eyed Seeing means 'learning to see from one eye with the strengths of Indigenous knowledges and ways of knowing, and from the other eye with the strengths of Western knowledges and ways of knowing and learning to use both these eyes together, for the benefit of all.' Marshall maintains that Etuaptmumk/Two-Eyed Seeing is a guiding principle, rather than a concept or theory. He states that it fosters the understanding that humanity cannot live within one perspective or one consciousness of the world (Canadian Encyclopaedia, 2026).

The collective work of Levac et al. (2018) recognizes that exploring links between Indigenous and Western knowledges may be contentious, however they go on to also suggest that with humility and respect, and as part of a broader conversation about the Calls to Action published by the Truth and Reconciliation of Canada (2012), there are opportunities to explore how these ideas might fit within our own positions and professional practices. Later in this chapter we will further unpack the idea of (cultural) humility vs (cultural) competency, where cultural competency and cultural humility are not synonymous. Competency suggests that learning is finite, if one is taught with the goal of being competent, the teaching concludes and one should possess the knowledge skills and abilities to respect and engage with various cultures. Cultural humility, on the other hand is a process of reflection and lifelong learning inquiry of personal and cultural biases as well as awareness and sensitivity to significant cultural issues of others (Yeager and Bauer-Wu, 2013).

The National Competency Framework for Paramedics (CSA, 2024) outline domains of activities that include (but are not limited to) person-centred care, safe care and professional care by paramedics. The Canadian Organization of Paramedic Regulators (COPR) have developed outcome statements for both paramedics and patients in the Canadian Paramedic Competency Framework (CPCF). COPR has also included specific statements related to competence and cultural safety and humility. Both the NCFP published by the CSA, and CPCF shared by COPR, will impact decisions that paramedics make about treatment of patients and their communities that is person centred, and culturally appropriate. Prior to development of the CPCF and NCFP many paramedic education programs were left using outdated guidance that included professional statements such as, 'maintain patient dignity' and 'identify cultural characteristics that impact patient dignity and acknowledge cultural differences'. This left a limited need perhaps to increase the level of taxonomy, using a verb like 'value' cultural differences and unpacking concepts that Elder Albert Marshall suggests, like Two-Eyed Seeing as a means of benefiting all in health and wellness.

In a taxonomy, learning objectives that address lower levels of learning are less complex and easier to achieve than are learning objectives at the upper levels of taxonomy (St Francis Xavier University, 2009). Herein begins an opportunity to unpack the need to increase the level of taxonomy with respect to cultural humility and person-centered care. Benjamin Bloom and his associates developed six taxonomies for the cognitive domain, that correlated with increasing level of difficulty (St Francis Xavier University 2009). The verb, identify, correlates to the first and lowest level taxonomy being the knowledge level. Conversely, a verb such as 'argue' would correlate with the highest-level taxonomy, the evaluation level. At this level of taxonomy, the learner develops an ability to make judgement or appraisals on knowledge or given criteria and use this judgement to guide their meaningful actions. The verb 'identify' and 'acknowledge' used in previous guidance (competency) profiles had an associated low-level taxonomy. Identify, would be synonymous with one's ability to memorize, to recall or otherwise repeat information presented earlier. This low level of taxonomy suggests little if any valuing the associated knowledge, skills or attitudes.

Let's bring back a few of those questions that opened this section. Have you ever wondered why so many family members are present at calls within the community to an indigenous home? Have you deliberately reflected on the patient and family's idea of wellness? It may depend. Were you taught to *identify* cultural differences or *value* person-centred care that may include Two-Eyed Seeing?

Making meaningful decisions that value person-centred care will include being curious and leaning into other's interpretations of what health and wellness means. One such example may come from indigenous beliefs that being surrounded by family and community and living in nature factor into 'feeling healthy'. Perhaps this provides insight into the number of family members present during a call to the home of an elder who is experiencing a traumatic event, or why you may experience smoke that is present from the ceremonial burning of sage during a smudging.

What we have learned and to what degree we have been able to learn concepts of health and wellbeing will depend on one's life experiences and the education provided to them on the subject. A lecture or powerpoint on diversity, equity and inclusion may not provide a learner with the opportunity to apply new knowledge skills or judgement into a developing professional practice. On the other hand, an immersive and interactive experience that involves interacting with a human with lived experience in a safe learning environment may allow for learners to practice humility and connecting with others who do not share similar life journeys. Perhaps consider what you have been taught as 'health and wellbeing' and consider the concept offered by Elder Albert Marshall on Two-Eyed Seeing and the opportunity we have to combine an Indigenous and Western understanding of wellbeing. We have hinted at being open to the idea of reflecting a few times. And this chapter will soon begin to talk about bias and the different types of biases and how they may impact decision making. Before we get to bias, we also need to introduce the idea of positionality.

Why is Positionality Important?

Positionality in life is important to appreciate and begins to inform inclusivity. Positionality begins to form some of the biases and interpretations of life around us and the lens through which we may feel things to be true. These interpretations, perspectives and reactions are socially constructed over the years.

Acknowledging positionality helps appreciate that others, will have their own perspectives and reactions that have been socially constructed and will be different from one person to the next. It is important for paramedics to lean into these different perspectives in hopes to provide true patient and family centred care.

Deciding to care may be impacted by one's positionality and may also include one's ability to connect with an individual, appreciating their positionality or their story and being curious about their perception of wellness. It has been suggested that 'if you cannot connect with people on a human level, if you cannot show that you care, if you cannot earn trust, your patients will suffer' (Stewart et al, 2024).

This decision to care is a decision that should surface not just from a theoretical or professional obligation nor regulatory requirement but rather a sincere desire to impact the wellness of another human. At the root of paramedicine, there ought to be a fundamental desire to care *about* people in addition to *for* people. When we care about people, our decisions that we make may be rooted in advocating for those same people.

It should be noted that positionality is not exclusively a patient-facing issue. Positionality also affects Indigenous paramedics and healthcare workers who may bring experiences of racism, intergenerational trauma, or systemic exclusion into their work.

Biases, both unconscious and conscious, can have a major impact on decision making and can make a difference to the quality of care that patients receive, as well as the patient outcomes they achieve in terms of their long-term physical and psychological health. This chapter will explore the decision-making and judgement processes, showing how biases can act as a barrier to effective and inclusive decision making. It will demonstrate how to best mitigate against bias and make our decisions more compassionate and inclusive as a result.

What Is Bias and Why Does It Happen?

Human beings are hardwired to be biased and we all have biases. Bias makes us inclined to favour some things and give them preference over others.

In-groups and Out-groups

There is a huge body of research that unsurprisingly confirms that we tend to feel more comfortable with people that are similar to us and who look like us. The concept of in-groups ('us') and out-groups ('them') is part of social identity theory, which was first established by psychologists Henri Tajfel and John Turner (1979). In-groups are those groups to which a person identifies as belonging and being accepted as part of. Out-groups are the opposite; these are groups to which a person does not belong. Out-group members can be singled out for their differences and discriminated against by members of an in-group. There are many groups to which a person may identify as belonging to, depending on how they categorize and make sense of their environment. Whether you see your patients as part of your in-group, or as outsiders and out-group members, may be a deciding factor as to how you treat them (Leaper, 2011).

System-1 and System-2 Thinking

As we know, System-1 thinking is largely considered to be automatic and unconscious, whereas System-2 thinking requires us to be present, pay attention to thought and be intentional in thinking.

Our preferences are shaped at an early age by socialization, our experiences and exposure to various societal mediums. To enable us to learn at speed, the brain makes quick connections to experiences of ideas and people from recollections that happened in the past. We use these preferences as filters by which to judge and make sense of the world. The categories can be activated by perceived characteristic identity such as gender, ethnicity, disability, sexual orientation, obesity, for instance.

Unfortunately, the brain's placement of information into categories in System-1 judgement is not always reliable. It may not be informed by fact or truth and further information gathering to validate or challenge beliefs and ideas is often not carried out. Lack of sleep, tiredness and overload of information can play an important role for the brain in deciding when System-1 and System-2 judgement and decision making is used. When we are tired the brain's tendency will be to use System-1 judgement as this type of decision making is an easier process for the brain and one where the brain does not have to consciously think. System-1 decision making can be helpful when it comes to mundane repetitive tasks such as cleaning your teeth or riding a bike. System-1 thinking contains memories that are deeply embedded in our brains. These are automatic processes where conscious thought is not required.

We can become over-reliant on System-1 thinking due to time pressures. System-1 thinking proved very useful to us in our evolutionary past, and we still rely on it now, to instinctively kick in to keep us safe when faced with dangerous situations.

Thousands of years ago, we used this kind of thinking to stop us from being eaten by predators whereas in the present day it is useful for assessing other dangers, such as being knocked down by traffic while crossing a busy road. The drawback is that when the more automatic, System-1 type of thinking is used to inform important decisions that affect patient care, it can have an impact on the quality of the care and the safety of the patient.

Unconscious Bias

'People that live with obesity are lazy, and they are to blame for their obesity', some people may think – or perhaps you may even assume this is true without realizing it. This is unconscious bias. Assumptions and stereotypes made to categorize a patient's identity, such as age, race, sexual orientation, religion, disability or gender could be down to unconscious bias. Patients you have a positive rapport with will often receive more of your time and attention, even though you may not consciously be aware of treating them any differently. Or perhaps you may relate to some patients in a particular manner because of the beliefs and stereotypes you might have about their ethnicity, disability, gender, culture, religious belief or sexual orientation. Of course, you might not have made these assumptions about these particular characteristics, but may still have made different assumptions of your own just like these.

Unconscious bias can affect how you view the patient and inform the decision that you make about their care, it causes us to value one group of people more highly than another group of people. This can create a hierarchy of care with some patients being treated more favourably than others and resulting in a worse experience and outcome for those patients whom we unconsciously, or even consciously, do not favour.

It is important to recognize that patients too may have unconscious biases. One example might include a patient asking to be treated by male paramedics, instead of female paramedics, because they believe that women are not as competent. Some patients may also exhibit unconscious racial bias and refuse treatment from paramedics who belong to an ethnic minority.

It is important that patients understand that it is not for them to choose who gives them care – just as paramedics cannot choose who they give care to and who they do not.

Conscious Bias

Conscious bias is the intentional and conscious choice to favour one group of people over another. Examples of conscious bias may include favouring men over women (sexism), favouring white people over people from ethnic minorities (racism), favouring able-bodied people over disabled people (ableism) or favouring heterosexual people over gay/lesbian, bisexual, transgender people (homophobia, biphobia and transphobia). Most people understand that this behaviour is against the law, that it is unacceptable behaviour and that it has no place in our society. Legislation such as the Equality Act 2010, Human Rights Act and the Public Sector Equality Duty, as well as organizational procedures and policies, are there to dissuade and deal with people who exhibit intentional prejudice and discrimination based on protected characteristics. Should a paramedic deliberately act on their prejudices to discriminate, they could face disciplinary action, a fitness to practise case, dismissal from employment or criminal proceedings.

How Can Bias Impact Decision Making?

Bias can result in incorrect treatment, poor outcomes and negative patient experience. It could even be the difference between life and death for some patients.

There is a requirement to minimize inequality in care. Research that took place in the USA into the influence of patient race on the administration of analgesia by student paramedics found that there was inequality of analgesia provision given based on race (Lord and Khalsa, 2019). The results revealed that African American patients were given less pain relief than white patients. A UK report published in March 2021 showed that implicit or unconscious bias can have a negative impact on decision making, and this may be worsened by societal responses to biased media reports, such as the use of the term 'the Chinese virus' used by some politicians when referring to Covid-19. The report looked at the differences among patients from different ethnic backgrounds, the degrees of severity the disease had, and the impact on patient outcomes (Gopal, 2021). The study also cites the 2019 report published by MBRRACE-UK, which highlighted the increase in maternal and perinatal mortality rates in pregnant black women (MBRRACE-UK, 2019), as well as discussing biases related to patients that suffer from obesity.

Recent research conducted in the USA into baby survival found that black newborns were more likely to survive childbirth when cared for by black doctors. The findings also found that black babies were three times more likely to die than white babies when cared for by white doctors (Greenwood et al., 2020). The research reveals the harmful consequences that bias can have on a patient's outcome. Although more research is required to fully understand the reasons for this outcome, it does highlight the importance of healthcare organizations' role in addressing bias and investigating the link to institutional racism to ensure equitable health outcomes for all.

How Can Paramedics Consider and Mitigate Against Bias Within Their Roles?

Although it is not possible to totally eradicate bias due to its innate condition, it may be possible to mitigate against it. Below are some actions that can be taken towards reducing bias.

Identifying Unconscious Bias

We like to believe in general that we are open minded, that we welcome difference and that we are not biased. Therefore, it can be really hard for us to identify our biases, especially as we can be unaware of them; they can be like blind spots. Harvard University developed the Implicit Association Test to measure unconscious bias; it is able to identify our unconscious bias through a number of tests (Project Implicit, 2011).

The tool is not perfect and has come under some criticism, particularly for its retest reliability in the same person and its highly specific contextualized nature. Nevertheless, this does not mean that the test has no merit. More research is required to better understand unconscious bias and its interrelationship with other matters that may impact the result. There is an innate complexity to measuring thought processes that sit outside of our consciousness; this complexity exists with most attitudinal and behavioural measures (FitzGerald et al., 2019). However, some people who have

> **Activity**
>
> Why not measure your unconscious bias?
>
> The Implicit Association Test can be found here: https://implicit.harvard.edu/implicit/takeatest.html

undertaken this test have reportedly found it a useful tool in revealing bias and giving the chance for reflection, heightened awareness of behaviour and an opportunity to address it.

Unconscious Bias Training

There has been much criticism of unconscious bias training by the UK government as having no impact on behaviour (Lopez, 2020). It is true that unconscious bias training does not necessarily change behaviour. However, it can also be argued that unconscious bias training was never set up to change behaviour. Its purpose is to increase awareness of the drivers of behaviour. It is important that we understand what is behind behaviours if we are to have any hope of trying to change them.

Unconscious bias training would need to sit alongside several other interventions and therefore, arguably, policy makers and professional bodies should consider making recommendations to update undergraduate curricula to reflect this need as an intrinsic aspect of core clinical education. There is good reason for unconscious bias training to be included on the paramedic science degree curriculum within the educational component about human factors. The Royal College of Paramedics recommends that human factors be incorporated in the paramedic science degree curriculum (College of Paramedics, 2024).

Being an Ally

An ally is someone who intentionally emphasizes and promotes inclusion through conscious action to benefit all. When a person with privilege works in conjunction with, and in support of, people from a marginalized group to amplify their voices, it is known as allyship. We all have the ability to be an ally within intersectional privilege. For example, a heterosexual person can be an ally to members of the 2SLGBTQ+ community, able-bodied people can be allies to disabled people, and men can be allies to women. Allies can take action to use their position of power, agency and influence to affect change.

Examples of how people can show allyship include educating themselves about different cultures and different lived experiences, and working to ensure that underrepresented voices are heard, included, appreciated and respected. It may include both small and big actions, such as speaking out when you see something is wrong or detrimental to marginalized groups. One aim is the acknowledgement, calling out and dismantling of systemic inequalities and unequal power structures for marginalized groups.

An ally can also enhance the culture of inclusion by engaging with their marginalized patients and colleagues and forming alliances with marginalized groups grounded in trust and accountability. Allies believe underrepresented people's lived experiences and worse outcomes. They hold themselves accountable and apologize when mistakes happen, as well as being prepared to adjust approaches towards allyship

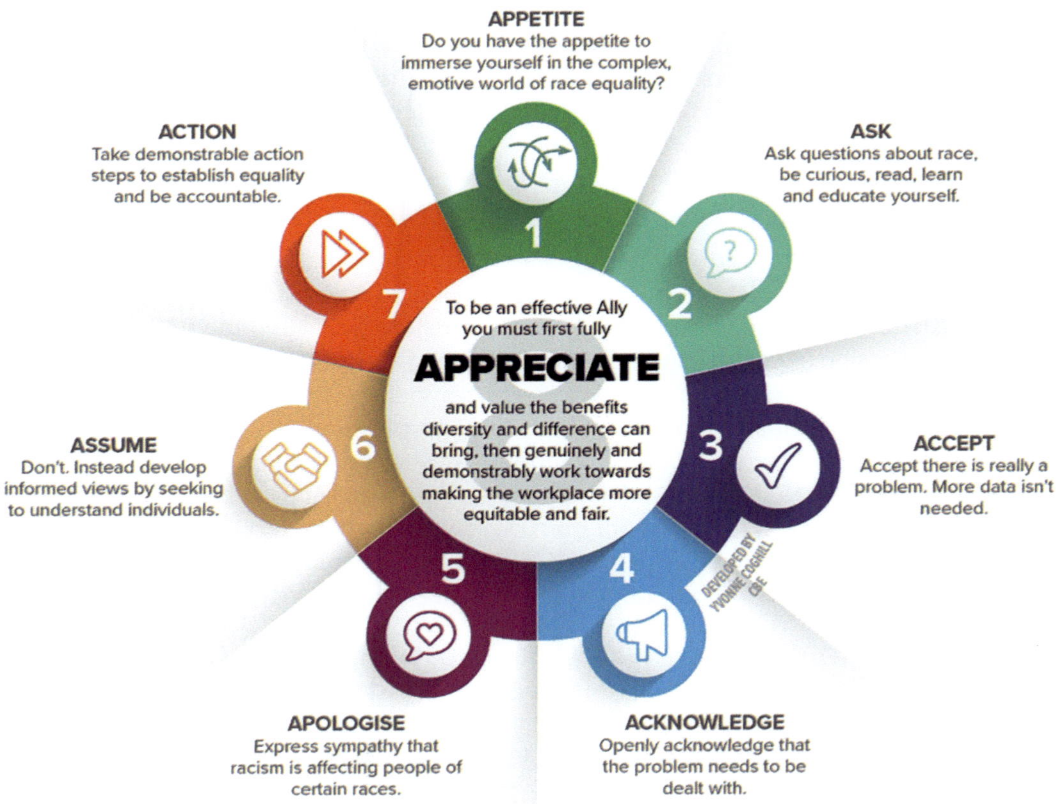
APPETITE
Do you have the appetite to immerse yourself in the complex, emotive world of race equality?
ACTION
Take demonstrable action steps to establish equality and be accountable.
ASK
Ask questions about race, be curious, read, learn and educate yourself.
1
2
7
To be an effective Ally you must first fully
APPRECIATE
and value the benefits diversity and difference can bring, then genuinely and demonstrably work towards making the workplace more equitable and fair.
6
3
ASSUME
Don't. Instead develop informed views by seeking to understand individuals.
ACCEPT
Accept there is really a problem. More data isn't needed.
5
4
DEVELOPED BY YVONNE COGHILL CBE
APOLOGISE
Express sympathy that racism is affecting people of certain races.
ACKNOWLEDGE
Openly acknowledge that the problem needs to be dealt with.

Figure 4.1 Eight As of authentic allyship.

Source: © Yvonne Coghill. Reproduced with kind permission.

when required. Allyship presents an opportunity for individuals to gain valuable insight and different perspectives so they can grow and learn about themselves and others.

Allyship can improve patient care as the clinician is proactive and intentional about understanding and embracing difference; this can then be reflected in the best quality, care and treatment that the patient receives. Empathy and synergy can be used to create a better patient experience. We know that when marginalized groups feel supported and included, they feel more comfortable in bringing their whole selves to a situation. This increases understanding, which means potential barriers between patient and clinician can be broken down, which creates opportunity for fuller engagement, inclusive decision making and better patient care and outcomes.

Allyship involves an investment of time to support and learn about others. The work of allyship is not about personal accolade and reward; it is about work and efforts being recognized by those groups that you wish to create change for. It is the lifelong journey of re-centring and understanding marginalized groups and the unequal power structure in society where some people are favoured over others.

Figure 4.1 describes eight attributes that are considered necessary for authentic allyship. This diagram shows how allyship supports racialized minorities, but can also be a useful reference for all allyship relationships including 2SLGBTQ+, disability and gender.

Moving from Cultural Competency to Cultural Humility

Cultural competency in healthcare consists of learning and demonstrating knowledge about patients' diverse backgrounds, including their values, belief systems, customs, traditions and feelings, and translating this into the patient's care. Cultural competency will also include understanding the individual's social and psychological requirements. In theory, cultural competency sounds like a good idea, but we must be careful that it does not lead to generalization and stereotyping of diverse groups. If the goal of cultural competency is to have cultural expertise, then we must ask ourselves if it is a realistic goal. Is it really possible to be truly competent and fluent in a culture that is different from our own? If we were to live in a country that was culturally different from our own, we could expect it to take a substantial amount of time to learn and be fluent in the customs and practice of the culture.

Comparatively, cultural humility, is about being culturally humble, and takes into consideration power dynamics. It is the lifelong journey of respecting and understanding difference to mitigate against the impact of bias. Cultural humility can be viewed as more of a transformational mindset and emphasizes that no culture is superior to any other.

Cultural humility is a continual process of learning, personal reflection, and acknowledging and being aware of one's own biases. It sits comfortably in the fact that mistakes may happen and from these mistakes there should be learning opportunities and reflection for ongoing improvement. It emphasizes being comfortable to ask if you are not sure about something. Cultural humility acknowledges that when learning about different cultures you may never fully understand everything about someone else's culture, and no-one gets it right all the time. It is about non-judgementally taking the perspective of the patient into consideration. Cultural humility allows both the paramedic and the patient to play an active role in the reduction of bias through active empathic learning and understanding. It allows for open discussion as well as accountability on the learning journey.

Cultural humility is a commitment to being curious and open to continuous learning of difference, and reflecting this in professional practice as knowledge and understanding are increased. Cultural humility is about having respect and due regard for different cultures; an example of this could be observing and understanding norms and practices of how different cultures may deal with death. Cultural competency gives the impression of a final destination of knowledge basis, whereas cultural humility shows appreciation for the process of continuous gathering of knowledge that can be used to inform and enhance practice as more knowledge and awareness is gleaned.

In 2015, the Truth and Reconciliation Commission of Canada published 94 Calls to Action. Within those calls to action, there are very specific actions related to the provision of education and healthcare. Examples of these calls to action within healthcare include:

- Measurable goals to identify and close the gaps in health outcomes between Aboriginal and non-Aboriginal communities
- Recognize, respect, and address the distinct health needs of the Métis, Inuit, and off-reserve Aboriginal peoples
- Recognize the value of Aboriginal healing practices.

There is also a very specific call to provide cultural competency training for all health-care professionals. Within the publication of both Paramedic Essential Regulatory Requirement documents and the National Competency Framework for Paramedics there is now language that supports the inclusion of cultural humility to exist within standards of care.

Since the Calls to Actions were published progress progress has been uneven, and healthcare remains an area where the gap between commitment and action is especially significant. For example 55 indigenous communities exist in Quebec, and only five have equitable access to EMS. The others are typically transported by private vehicle in less-than-adequate situations. Clinicians should get used to questioning decisions and conclusions as well as challenging themselves and colleagues about each other's assumptions and stereotypes (Khan, 2021).

Psychological Safety

People need to feel comfortable to speak up and raise concerns in situations where they are aware of bias directed at the patient or if they experience it themselves. Team members need to feel safe and comfortable to share their concerns; this includes views that may not be congruent with the majority view. People keep back their views for many reasons including fear of conflict with peers or challenging senior staff. Open cultures and safe environments need to be created in order for paramedics to feel free and able to speak up and be heard (Delizonna, 2017).

Metacognition

Metacognition is practising awareness of one's thought processes and understanding the patterns (or bias) behind them. It can provide useful insight into your own thinking. It is mainly used in learning and education.

Metacognition encourages self-questioning of a person's own knowledge in order to direct their thinking and determine the support they may need. It also encourages using discourse to examine ideas with peers. This helps to identify gaps in knowledge, as well as learning from and gaining other people's insight. The kind of questions that individuals might ask are:

- What went well?
- What could I have done better?
- If it is good practice, can this be replicated and used in different situations?

Slowing Down the Thought Process

Daniel Kahneman advocates for the slowing down of the 'quick fire' thought process of System 1 mentioned earlier in this chapter. Allowing for the transfer of the System-1 thought process to System-2 causes an intentional delinking so that System-1 thought processes can be verified, with data and facts analysed, for better-informed decision making (Kahneman, 2012). Important to note, as mentioned elsewhere in the book, there are times when we have to think fast based on very obvious cues, such as haemorrhage or cardiac arrest.

A trial looking at antibiotic prescribing found that changes in working practice that made clinicians slow down during the prescription process and contemplate 'why' and 'how' they were prescribing had a positive effect. Comments from the qualitative analysis suggested that the slowed-down process reminded them to think about important matters that they may not otherwise have thought about, and steered them towards deliberate and reasoned thinking (O'Sullivan, 2018; Jones et al., 2017).

Two Brains Are Better Than One

Encouraging diversity within teams can help reduce bias. A Harvard Business Review article states that 'diverse teams are more likely to constantly re-examine facts and remain objective. They may also encourage greater scrutiny of each member's actions, keeping their joint cognitive resources sharp and vigilant' (Rock and Grant, 2016). A diverse team can aid mitigation against the risks of bias in treating patients from diverse backgrounds. A few suggestions on how paramedic teams can encourage diversity are listed below:

- Attraction of diversity to the team.
- A team environment where people are encouraged and feel psychologically safe to bring their whole selves to work.
- A team culture where all members of the team feel a sense of belonging and that they have a voice that matters and is heard.
- Ensuring that every team member is valued for their difference, individual skills and abilities.
- Encouraging all team members to be open to hearing difference of thought and opinion.

Intentionally Diversify Your Network

By intentionally connecting and actively seeking out exposure to people from different backgrounds and experiences than yourself, individuals can enrich their learning and acceptance of difference. This could be done by attending community events, reading books, listening to podcasts, watching films by diverse authors or covering relevant subjects, or even trying out different foods. It might be hoped that these practices in time could help us to embrace difference instead of seeing difference as 'other' and classifying people in out-groups.

Reciprocal Mentoring

In many organizations reciprocal mentoring is now being practised and benefits gained. This is where people from under-represented groups (such as black, Asian or other marginalized ethnicities, 2SLGBTQ+, disability) are paired with people from majority groups in an equal two-way relationship. Through conversation with each other they share their knowledge and lived experiences. Purposeful conversation and an exchange of insights can contribute to enhanced awareness, increased perspectives, and greater empathy and understanding of each other. This can directly contribute towards the creation of more equitable and inclusive decision making. Reciprocal mentoring has been found to be a safe space where factors that may cause inequity can be positively explored and proactively addressed. This practice can be a powerful driver for change, challenging mindsets and enriching thought processes through conversation. Individuals usually meet once a month for a duration of 6 months.

These conversations are yielding positive results in increasing knowledge and dismantling barriers. A field experiment was undertaken in the USA involving a door-to-door canvassing intervention to combat anti-transgender prejudice. It proved that a single approximately 10-minute conversation actively taking the perspective of others can markedly reduce prejudice for at least a 3-month period (Broockman and Kalla, 2016).

Communication Skills

Many of the actions for mitigating bias in this chapter centre around the notion that clear communication can help to decrease bias thinking and increase positive outcomes: understanding, empathy and open-mindedness. This is by no means a novel idea; strong interpersonal communication skills are essential in ensuring that paramedics provide high quality, effective and safe clinical practice. Effective communication can have a positive effect on the patient's physical and emotional state with better outcomes and satisfaction for the patient.

Paramedics are required to work and communicate effectively and professionally with their colleagues, other healthcare professionals and patients. They can often find themselves in very stressful and critical situations. Poor communication can result in the wrong decisions being made about a patient's care and can have devastating consequences, which could result ultimately in death.

Communication not only covers communication with the patient who requires medical care, but also communication with work colleagues, teams and hospital staff that the patient is being transferred on to. Paramedics must be able to connect with the patient quickly to establish good rapport and put the patient at ease, and to obtain relevant information in order to give the highest possible quality of care.

It could be reasoned that effective communication for paramedics is just as important as the medicine that is administered to patients. The World Health Organization (2009) highlights communication as being one of the most crucial elements of patient safety. The WHO stated some of the key problems relating to communication were the following: shift or patient handovers; the quality of information recorded in patient files, case notes and incident reports; status effects inhibiting junior staff from speaking up; and difficulties of transmitting information within and between organizations.

The Leonard, Graham and Bonacum (2004) study found that communication failure accounted for 70% of sentinel events. Similarly, the Joint Commission report (2008) cited by Dingley et al. (2012) showed that communication failure is the third highest factor for sentinel deaths, behind this are leadership and human factors (Dingley et al., 2012). These studies emphasize the importance of clear communication, as it really can be the difference between life and death.

The Elements of Communication

Traditionally, the necessary elements of communication are:

A sender – person sending a message to another person.

A channel – the means by which the message is conveyed.

A receiver – person receiving the message.

The traditional elements given are based on the principles of the Shannon-Weaver model of communication. Noise is also referred to in this model and is interpreted as being something that may distort or stop the message being conveyed in the way that the sender had intended.

During human communication, a person has to either code or decode a message. The simple ways of coding messages are to put them into language, which is either speech or writing and/or non-verbal communication, for example, body language. The receiver then decodes the words and non-verbal signals by interpreting the message to understand the true intention and meaning behind it that the sender is wanting the recipient to receive and understand. The Shannon-Weaver communication model (n.d.) has been further added to, broadening its scope to include checking the understanding of the message and feedback incorporating the cyclic holistic nature of communication, rather than portraying it as only being a linear process. The feedback loop in communication is of importance in stressful incidents or when communicating information that may not be easy to understand or have a degree of complexity, such as, such as a medical history. It is essential that the correct communication has not only been received but is thoroughly understood, leaving no room for misinterpretation and the consequences that this may bring.

Within the context of paramedicine, the goal of communication is to receive and convey information in a way that results in the best care and outcome for the patient. When we think of communication, most of the time we might only think about one element – speech. We can forget that listening is an essential component of communication. Research suggests that adults spend approximately 70% of their time communicating; this breaks down on average as 45% listening, 30% speaking, 16% reading and 9% writing (Adler et al., 2001).

To be an active listener and communicate well is a much-needed skill for paramedics. First, we must hear what patients are saying to us to be able to help them. It is essential that paramedics are able to quickly develop a rapport and create a space that encourages hearing what patients and families are saying.

Verbal Communication

Verbal communication can be divided into two broad areas (Blaber, 2008): language and vocabulary and paralinguistic features.

Language and Vocabulary

As a paramedic there will be times when you will need to adjust your language and vocabulary to suit the situation and person that you are communicating with. For instance with other healthcare professionals, you may need to express and convey more complex medical terms and professional language. Misunderstanding can most often occur between paramedics and patients when a common language is not shared. With patients you may be required to adjust your communication to suit

Tips to Ensure Clear Communication

- Avoid saying too much all in one go; people can only process a limited amount of new information at a time, and this is particularly true in stressful situations.
- Speak concisely and clearly.
- Check to see whether your communication is being understood as you have intended by the patient/recipient.
- Be conscious and put thought into what you want to say and the delivery.
- Be aware of your communication style.

their needs, for instance, simplifying language where the patient possesses a limited range of language, such as a patient whose additional language is English and their fluency is impacted. Support with language translation can also be accessed. Adjustments to communication may also be required for children or those with cognitive impairment, such as dementia patients, those with learning difficulties and those with a sensory disability, such as a hearing impairment.

Paralinguistic

The way that something is said, the tone and manner in which it is said, can be just as important as what is said and can impact how the communication is received and understood. Paralinguistic is an essential component of non-verbal communication. It comprises pitch, tone, volume, emotion and speaking method. It can let the receiver of the communication know whether there is interest or lack of it. Dr Albert Mehrabian, a behavioural psychologist researching body language, separated out the components of communication. His research found that communication was 7% words only, 38% vocal and 55% non-verbal (Mehrabian, 1981). It is important to recognize that the formula applies to the communication of feelings and attitudes.

Examples of non-verbal communication include:

- Facial expression
- Eye contact
- Gesture and posture
- Personal space and touch.

When thinking about forms of communication, it is important that they are appropriate for the situation. For example, when gathering a history from a patient, it is important that they are the centre of your attention; patients should feel connected and have enough trust to give you key information. Making eye contact, head nodding and acknowledging their communication with small verbal gestures such as 'OK' and 'yes' as they are speaking, can encourage someone to communicate effectively with you. This encouragement is known as active listening. Through active listening people are usually more likely to continue communicating and reveal all the information you need in order to assess them properly.

Equally, you should observe the body language of those you are communicating with; it can give you further information about that person's feelings and needs, and enable you to prepare an appropriate response. For example, you may be able to tell from someone's body language if they are feeling angry or frustrated. Your observation of their body language could then give you the option to change your method of communication in your response to one that might de-escalate the situation.

The Importance of Communication with Each Other

It matters greatly how we communicate with our colleagues and other medical and healthcare professionals. Providing excellent patient care requires excellent teamwork. We know that teams that function and communicate well outperform dysfunctional teams and make for better patient outcomes.

It will come as no surprise that the research shows that for high functioning teams communication is key, and they perform better, which leads to better patient outcomes. Medical teams perform worse when confronted with rudeness, as documented by the charity Civility Saves Lives:

> Riskin and Erez demonstrated the negative impact of rudeness on clinical outcomes. They conducted a Randomized Control Trial using resus scenarios comparing one with rudeness within the team to without. Their research showed that when rudeness was present, there was an increase in diagnostic and procedural errors, and they were able to attribute more than 50% of this to the rudeness.
>
> (Civility Saves Lives, n.d.; citing Risken et al., 2015).

Written Communication

Every patient contact will normally involve a form of written communication. This will usually be notes (paper or electronic) for the completion of the patient record. Keeping up-to-date, accurate patient clinical records is part of a paramedic's role. The notes will be reviewed to inform medical opinion by other healthcare professions. Written information can more easily be understood if it follows a logical format and is concise and legible.

Excessive use of shorthand can be hard for another clinician to subsequently follow and understand. Medical terminology can often be condensed to acronyms, and this can act as a barrier to communication between clinicians. It is therefore important that paramedics are trained and have a full understanding of medical terminology and acronyms.

Social and Cultural Context

Communication relies heavily on the social and cultural context. We are in control of how we wish to communicate information. What we are not in control of is how individuals will engage with the received information. Some recipients may actively avoid certain information or information that triggers an emotional reaction. Their response to information can be shaped by their social and cultural contexts, which may be different from yours, as well as their own needs for psychological safety and the extent to which they trust the source and the person giving the information.

As a paramedic you will be required to ensure that you communicate as well as possible when using verbal and non-verbal communication to ensure that it is received in the manner that you intend. Every day, you will meet people from a wide range of social and cultural backgrounds. Every one of these people inhabits a different social or cultural context, and you will need to be mindful of modifying your communication, based on the needs of the individual and respect for their diverse cultural or social backgrounds, to ensure that accurate messages are passed on and confusion is avoided.

Challenges to Communication

Challenges to effective communication can exist on the part of the patient/family member or the healthcare professional. These challenges can take many forms, for example, patients who have a sensory impairment, such as a hearing or sight impairment. However, there are simple strategies to use, such as ensuring patients have any supporting aids, such as hearing aids or glasses.

One of the barriers to a paramedic's effective communication is being unaware of the plan of care. Best practice includes the recognition of any existing care plans. This is to ensure that the paramedic is able to take the plan into consideration as a means of informing their own decision making and ensuring that their future care instruction is aligned with the plan.

Pain can be an enormous challenge to effective communication, and can be the cause of patient fearfulness, confusion and distress. There are two useful frameworks that have been developed to support healthcare professionals in acknowledging and resolving effective communication. The first is represented by the acronym FEARS (fears, environment, attitudes, responses, skills) (Table 4.1), and the second by the acronym FIBS (fears, inadequate skills, beliefs, support) (Table 4.2) (Nicol and Nyatanga, 2017).

Improving Communication Awareness

Self-assessment of interpersonal communication skills can be used as a tool in identifying strengths and weaknesses. Second year paramedic students from

Table 4.1 FEARS: Potential Patient Challenges to Communication

FEARS Element	Manifestation
Fears	Being judged as ungrateful; being stigmatized; crying/breaking down; burdening/causing distress to the health professional
Environment	Lack of privacy; person present or absent who needs to be/not be there with me
Attitudes	This person does not have time to listen to me, or it is not this person's job to talk about this; my concerns are not important; I should be able to cope with this; my family would not want me to talk about this
Responses (from healthcare professionals)	Distanced or disengaged; relevant questions were not asked of me; being touched when I need my own space
Skills	I cannot find the right words/have not sufficient command of language/do not understand enough to know what to ask; literacy levels; mental capacity issues

Source: Nicol and Nyatanga, 2017

Table 4.2 FIBS: Potential Challenges to Communication

FIBS Element	Manifestation
Fears	Causing upset or harm; emotional responses; saying 'the wrong thing'; being asked difficult questions; taking too much time
Inadequate skills	Lack of assessment skills for psychological issues and concerns as well as physical ones; inability to integrate physical and non-physical agenda together into a full holistic review
Beliefs	Emotional problems are inevitable in serious/life-threatening illness, nothing can be done about them so it is pointless to bring up issues we 'cannot solve'; it is 'someone else's role to do this'
Support	Lack of support for the patient if problems are identified; feeling professionally unsupported; team conflicts

Source: Nicol and Nyatanga, 2017

Monash University, Australia, took part in research to identify their perceptions of their interpersonal communication competence. An assessment of their perceptions of their interpersonal communication skills was measured using the Interpersonal Communication Competence Scale (ICCS). The results revealed that student paramedics reported their interpersonal communication skills as being high, but their skills in areas that related to assertiveness and listening skills as lower. It was a small sample size, and it is acknowledged that further research may be of benefit with larger sample sizes (Ross et al., 2014). Managerial structures, such as one-to-one meetings, appraisals and clinical supervision, are a good opportunity for paramedics to receive feedback concerning interpersonal and communication skills. Feedback from patients and colleagues through surveys, compliments and complaints is another source of useful feedback. All feedback can increase a person's self-awareness of their communication strengths and weaknesses, identifying where improvement is required and the adjustments that may be needed.

Culture and Ethnicity: The Impact on Disease Manifestations and Effect on Health Outcomes

There is no doubt that if clinicians were more familiar with the differences in presentations of serious urgent and emergency conditions in people of different ethnic minorities, that this would improve patient care, reduce health inequity and save lives. There have been cases of specific conditions, which have resulted in serious incidents and even deaths, when they have not been recognized early enough by clinicians.

Reducing inequity in care for people with darker skin tones may include the following topics:

- **Recognizing anaemia/pallor:** We can ask the patient to turn their palms to face the ceiling, there may be reduced darkness in the creases of the palms; this is not a very accurate sign so cannot be used on its own, and other information should also be considered. We can also compare the colour of the patient's palms with that of a family member or look at the conjunctiva, which may appear pale pink or white in anaemia, no matter what the person's skin colour.
- **Recognizing cyanosis**: Cyanosis can also be seen on the tongue and other areas inside the mouth; the blue-ish/grey discolouration may also be seen in the hands or feet, with or without the blue-ish discolouration in or around the lips and mouth. It is more difficult to detect in darker skin and may be most obvious when looking at the nails. After giving oxygen the patient's tongue and lips will revert to having a healthy pink colour and facial skin will appear the usual colour, not the 'ashen' (pale grey or blue-ish) tone associated with cyanosis.
- **Presentations of pain:** Consider conscious and unconscious biases in the assessment and clinical management of pain.

- **Recognizing bruising** (particularly in children and other vulnerable patients): Look carefully for fading bruises in people with dark skin, and ask the patient if they have any bruises. It may be difficult to see very recent bruising (which would appear red in people with lighter skin tones), and this might only become obvious as the colour of the bruising develops into a dark purple, brown or black, which is then darker than the surrounding skin. Also, the yellow discolouration of older bruises may be more subtle in darker skin tones. Bruising might be caused by bleeding disorders, medicines or non-accidental injuries. Some conditions may appear similar to bruising (e.g., Mongolian blue spots in children under the age of 4), and it is important to also recognize these as normal in some racial groups.
- **Death and End of Life Care:** In addition to pain management, consider if you are aware of differences between diverse groups in care around the end of life.
- **Recognition of the presentations of sickle cell disease and sickle cell crisis.**
- **Presentation of heart attacks:** Be aware of the different presentations in groups of patients who are not white males, including in black, Asian and racially minoritized patients, or women.
- **Pregnancy**:
    - Pain in relation to pregnancy and labour/birth – the importance of recognizing and adequately managing pain in all women.
    - Prevalence of tilted pelvis in black, Asian and racially minoritized women, and specific childbirth complications related to different groups of women.

Case Study

by Robert Bonspeil

The Call

It's late afternoon in early fall. The air is cool and the leaves are starting to turn. The call comes in from a house on a small First Nations community, and one unit is dispatched. The nearest hospital is about 40 to 45 minutes away depending on the road.

Marie and Derek are sent out for a 67-year-old man, Thomas. Dispatch notes are vague: 'not himself … not talking much.' When they pull up, there are already a couple of vehicles in the driveway. The front door is open.

Thomas's daughter, Sarah, meets them before they knock. She looks worried but composed.She keeps it simple: 'He's just … off. Couple days now. Not eating much. Sleeping a lot. This morning, he didn't make sense for a bit.'

Then she adds, more firmly: 'He doesn't want to go to the hospital.'

A pause, then quieter: 'He lost his brother there a few years back. Ever since … he doesn't trust it.'

Inside the House

The house is warm from a woodstove. Marie and Derek smell it as soon as they walk in. Thomas is sitting in a chair with a blanket over his legs. Two other family members are nearby. One older woman sits slightly off to the side, quiet but clearly paying attention to everything. There is some sage on the windowsill.

Thomas looks up when Marie and Derek enter. He makes brief eye contact, then drops his gaze. A moment later, he glances toward the older woman before settling back into silence.

Assessment

Derek starts. He is doing exactly what he was trained to do. He crouches in front of Thomas and begins with the usual questions:

- 'Can you tell me your name?'
- 'Do you know where you are?'
- 'What day is it?'

No response. Derek glances toward Sarah.

'Is this normal for him?' he asks.

There is a slight shift in the room. Nothing obvious, but it is there.

Marie steps in quietly. She does not rush. She pulls up a chair and sits beside Thomas instead of standing over him.

'Kwe, Thomas,' she says. 'Thanks for letting us come in.'

Thomas looks at her again. Same brief eye contact, but he doesn't turn away as quickly this time.

Marie turns slightly toward the older woman.

'Looks like you've all been watching over him,' she says, speaking to her but loud enough for everyone to hear.

A few nods around the room. Marie gives a small, respectful nod, then turns back to Thomas.

'Your family's worried about you. We just want to understand what's going on. You okay with that?'

He pauses, then nods.

After a few seconds, he speaks. He says he is tired and his legs feel heavy. There's no pain. He's just worn out.

Findings

They continue, slower this time.

- Glucose: 19.2 mmol/L
- Blood pressure: 148/92
- Breathing slightly laboured
- Dry mouth and reduced skin turgor

Thomas admits he has not been drinking much. On its own, its nothing dramatic. But put together, it is concerning.

The Decision

Marie explains what she is seeing in plain terms.

'This could be your sugar running high and your body drying out a bit. It can creep up on people.'

She does not push him.

'What are you thinking you'd like to do?' she asks.

Thomas takes his time. He looks down, then towards the older woman again. She gives a small, almost imperceptible nod.

Then he says: 'I'll go ... but she's coming with me.'

He nods toward Sarah.

Marie answers right away: 'Yeah. We can do that.'

The room shifts. You can feel it. They get him ready without rushing.

What Does This Show?

Clinically, this looks like hyperglycemia with dehydration. It could become serious if it is not addressed. But that is not what determines how the call goes.

Thomas was not being difficult. He was in his home, with unfamiliar people, being questioned right away.

Derek did nothing wrong, but he treated it like any other call.

This wasn't any other call.

Marie did not make a show of anything. She greeted him in his own language. She took a moment. She acknowledged the right person in the room, the elder, and spoke in a way that fit the space. She kept the family part of the conversation from the start. That was enough.

She gave Thomas time. She let the decision come from him, with his family. Respect. That matters.

Losing someone in a hospital is not just background information. In a small community, that kind of experience carries weight. If you ignore it, people shut down. If you respect it, they work with you. That is the difference between pushing someone onto a stretcher and having them walk out the door with you.

Reflection Points

- Avoid saying too much all in one go; people can only process a limited amount of new information at a time, and this is particularly true in stressful situations.
- Speak concisely and clearly.
- Check to see whether your communication is being understood as you have intended by the patient/recipient.
- Be conscious and put thought into what you want to say and the delivery.
- Be aware of your communication style.

    - Recognition and reporting of FGM and complications with childbirth.

- **Mental health presentations:** Consideration of conscious and unconscious bias in the assessment of people presenting in mental health crises.

We need to continue to look for more evidence and education for clinicians in order to minimize inequity in clinical care and ensure that in the future all clinicians and student clinicians can effectively assess and treat people from all the diverse communities for which we provide urgent and emergency care.

Conclusion

We can see that reducing the negative impact of bias is not an easy task and requires a multi-prong approach with various interrelated strategies. However, we know by trying to address bias, considering your understanding of health and wellness and being aware of your positionality, we can yield positive rewards and results for us as individuals and has the opportunity of improving the quality of care that we provide our patients, by making it more culturally sensitive and person centred. This can in turn enhance paramedics' practice and enable a better understanding of the diverse communities that they serve. We hope that this, in turn, will help to support and encourage better inclusive decision making.

Reflective Exercises

1. Imagine you were asked to assess a 4-year-old boy with a darker skin tone who had been non-specifically unwell and a bit 'grizzly'. The mother does not speak much English and the child is sleeping and more settled after some acetaminophen when you arrived. How carefully would you try to assess the child? Could you be confident you would not miss an early meningococcal rash? What system would you use to try to get as clear a history as possible;

would you rely on other family members including older children, or use a translation system? How might that impact on the outcome for the child?

2. Consider the impact of tiredness and how often you use System-1 or System-2 thinking at the start and end of a long shift. How aware are you of the impact of tiredness on clinical decision making and bias? How could you improve this to the benefit of your patients?
3. Think of a time you provided care as part of a team or crew for a patient from a different background from yours. Was the care to the same standard as for a patient from a similar background to yours? Did you feel confident to speak up if the care was inadequate? Were there any biases either conscious or unconscious from you, another clinician or from the patient or someone with them?
4. Consider a case you have seen with a woman in her 40s who presented with non-traumatic chest discomfort and anxiety, with a normal ECG. How did you manage this patient, was it the same as a man with a similar presentation who described a 'tight belt around my chest'?
5. Consider how you act as an ally to others. Make a list of the diverse groups of people you work with and care for, how for each group you actively seek to understand how they may face discrimination as well as conscious or unconscious bias, and how you would support them or challenge his.

Chapter 5

The Evolution of the Paramedic as a Critical Thinker

Andy Collen

Chapter objectives

This chapter will cover:

- Critical thinking in everyday life and in paramedic practice
- Values-based decision making and healthcare practice
- Information processing
- Barriers to critical thinking
- Intuition and experience in critical thinking
- Decision point management: taking control at each stage
- Summing up: moving from 'what' to 'why'.

Caution!

This chapter will introduce the process of challenging yourself in terms of what you believe when making decisions, and this process needs time and deliberation (System-2 thinking) (Kahneman, 2012). In paramedic practice, there are often situations where immediate action is required. It is this ability – among the wider skill set of paramedics – which helps define what paramedics do for patients in high-pressure situations.

The intention of this chapter, and those following, is to support the reader to develop a decision-making acumen that promotes better outcomes, but care must be taken to avoid delaying treatment when there is not the time to deliberate (System-1 thinking) (Kahneman, 2012). Do not let these new concepts prevent you from acting decisively in an emergency.

Critical Thinking in Everyday Life and Paramedic Practice

We covered the idea of bias in the last chapter. As human beings go through life, we may impose on ourselves (or accept) concepts that we believe to be true, accurate and correct. Whether this is a subjective opinion on what colours we consider to be appealing, or objective views that may or may not be factually correct, we tend to favour one thing over another for a variety of reasons. This is part of having a human personality.

Sharing views and opinions helps us form and maintain relationships. For example, supporting a particular football team (regardless of how often they lose) enables us to feel part of a group. The wide variety of factors that joins tribes together also has the power to divide, as our preferences in areas such as values, morals, ethics and tolerance are often highly subjective. Where decisions are left unchallenged, and never subject to reflection, they can become entirely intuitive. Or they can be based on cultural beliefs or tribal behaviours, and the level of influence or bias entirely missed. Some subjective tribal beliefs are harmless, but others lead to decisions being made that may be highly unethical (see Bioethics in Chapter 2, pp. 38–53, as well as Inclusive Decision Making in Chapter 4). The following example highlights an extreme instance of human vulnerabilities in thought and decision making, where **groupthink** and influence are strong.

Example: Vaccine Sceptics

The years 2020 through to 2022 (and possibly beyond) will be defined by the Covid-19 pandemic. The response to the global crisis led to rapid changes in treatments based on the developing understanding of the disease and the way in which it manifests. More incredible was the rapid development of the vaccines that became available for administration within a year of the genomic profile of the virus being mapped. The rapidity of this development led to some fearing the vaccine, and subsequently conspiracy theories developed.

Healthcare is a branch of science, and its membership (healthcare professionals) are able to review evidence and critically appraise information that is published about interventions, such as vaccines. Some members of wider society, possibly influenced by factors such as the MMR vaccine scandal, where Andrew Wakefield erroneously linked the measles, mumps and rubella (MMR) vaccine with the development of autism in children, have developed a collective suspicion of the new vaccines (Health Foundation, 2010).[1] Social media, buoyed by some elements of the press and popular culture, promoted views from some quarters that included theories about the vaccine, including notions of them containing nano-bots and having mind control components, through to more

[1] **N.B.** It is important to note that this section is intended to use a healthcare example to illustrate the point being made and no inference should be taken as to the very real and legitimate reasons why not all people elect to receive vaccinations.

basic safety concerns associated with the speed of development of the vaccine itself being disproportionate to the background risks associated with vaccines or any new drug relative to their benefits (Pertwee et al., 2022).

While personal choice is important when considering any medical intervention, the contagion against the vaccine is an example of groupthink in action. The anxiety created by the claims made, akin to those made in the MMR scandal, played on fear of the unknown and allowed a narrative to develop, which strengthened as the word spread. Of course, many people were also cautious about the vaccine for very valid reasons, such as known allergies, or cultural beliefs.

Publications from high impact journals (e.g., *The Lancet*, *British Medical Journal*, *Science*) based on robust scientific evidence may have little influence or acceptance among the anti-vaccine movement, and this has the potential to cause vaccine hesitancy or scepticism among those who may have previously accepted vaccines at face value. On the other hand, many of us consider the human and economic impact of a vaccination programme, compared with the realistic likelihood of a coordinated global movement to control people's minds (mindful that much of the propaganda is spread via social media apps on smart phones, devices that track your movements and record and share your preferences). Brandolini's law is an internet adage from 2013, which argues that there is increased effort needed to correct misinformation in comparison to the effort needed to instil it in the first place (Brandolini, 2013). As Mark Twain said, 'How easy it is to make people believe a lie, and how hard it is to undo that work again' (Griffin and Smith, 2013).

Illogical or intractable viewpoints are by no means unique in human history. It demonstrates that human beings are capable of being externally manipulated or even becoming blinkered to the wider ranges of choice and judgement, and some are prone to being influenced and misled into adopting narrow and flawed beliefs that are wildly at odds with the critical thinking of the majority of members of society. Consider the Stanford University experiment undertaken in 1971, where students adopted randomly assigned roles as either prisoners or guards. Within six days, the experiment was abandoned due to the behaviours of the 'guards' – students who only a few days previously were mild-mannered young undergraduates (Zimbardo et al., 1971). The prevailing culture provided a snapshot of how humans can react if the social norms are interrupted, and groupthink becomes established. These were intelligent people, and it is fascinating to reflect on how quickly the landscape changed and how reasonable decisions stopped being made. How can the culture in healthcare settings affect how we make decisions? Do we have 'bad apples' or 'bad barrels'?

> *How we went about testing these questions and what we found may astound you. Our planned two-week investigation into the psychology of prison life had to be ended after only six days because of what the situation was doing to the college students who participated. In only a few days, our guards became sadistic and our prisoners became depressed and showed signs of extreme stress.*
>
> (Professor Philip G. Zimbardo in Haney et al., 1973)

The links between these examples and patient care and clinical practice may seem distant, but there may be some aspects to your practice that you consider normal and mundane, and for which you have never been challenged. These may actually be quite outdated, outmoded or dangerous, and may have arisen through subliminal learning or within a small social group, manifested as groupthink or tribal behaviour. The examples given serve to illustrate that deeply rooted beliefs about what is correct or accurate may have been imparted in such a way that they may never be challenged. This is part of the human condition, so we do need to broaden our horizons in order to learn, reflect and make decisions. In the healthcare setting this takes on even greater level of importance as the ever evolving and developing evidence base means that challenging preconceptions is vital in preventing harm to patients.

The fact is that we are all capable of being influenced into unreasonable, irrational thoughts, acts and beliefs. Most are not harmful but are equally irrational – such as buying lottery tickets, fear of flying regardless of the prevailing statistics, or voluntarily listening to Coldplay (sorry, but I did say we are prone to subjectivity). The important principle of challenging preconceptions may, in the healthcare setting, alter some outcomes for the better for patients. Looking at the way humanity can be so easily influenced is important to highlight that we can all make poor decisions where we fail to critically appraise information and instead allow ourselves to 'go with the flow'. We will now try to understand why this happens, in the hope of ensuring it doesn't happen to us.

Values-based Decision Making and Healthcare Practice

As previously discussed, we are not inherently driven to constantly question ourselves, although this varies by our values and insights, and our appetite to adapt. This means that we can easily become entrenched in our ways and views. Regardless of this, these factors combine to form us as a person – for better or worse. The beliefs and experiences we accumulate, along with knowledge and learned behaviours, coalesce to become our personality. This works very nicely for the most part. Friendships are made on the basis of commonality of thought and purpose; values are defined and reinforced, and ultimately what we believe is true becomes as everyday as the impulse to reach for the light switch when you walk into a darkened room.

Critical thinking is a process for challenging, where appropriate and/or necessary, these entrenched truths – the **heuristically** implanted notions (mental shortcuts) that are stored as fact, but which can betray you – leading to a place where subjectivity can be replaced with objectivity where necessary. Clearly, this works best where something is equivocal rather than an opinion that has limited impact on others. For example, some people are moved by certain pieces of modern art and sculpture, while others think they are just piles of bricks or unmade beds. The point is that it doesn't really matter in that case as the subjectivity (in the form of an opinion) requires no establishment of fact and the beauty is, of course, in the eye of the beholder. When this is transferred to a health encounter, any subjectivity which is not robustly tested may be actively harmful, and this is in essence the cornerstone of evidence-based medicine (NICE, 2024). Imagine, for example, if you decided to assume that all children's rashes were caused by a simple viral infection, rather than a bacterial illness, and refused to examine any evidence that might contradict this. If your diagnostic preference went unchallenged, it would ultimately lead to poor outcomes for some patients. The basis of what we observe or test for as clinicians should be treated with suspicion and doubt until it can be reduced to fact (or as near to fact as possible). We will now look at the process of turning 'what' to 'why', and how following this mantra can provide a really simple method for ensuring that each encounter you have with patients is approached in such a way as to ensure you can test your skills and knowledge and come up with the best answer for the presentation you are facing.

Exercise: Turning WHAT into WHY

Please look at the image below.

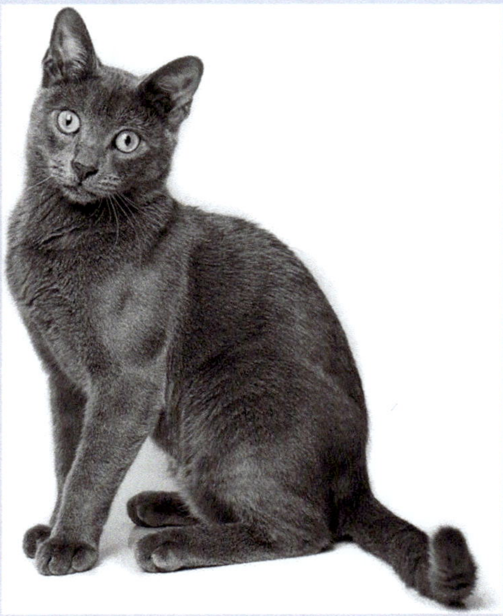

Figure 5.1 Object identification.

Can you identify the subject of Figure 5.1? Of course, you can, but all you have done is say 'what' it is. Now look again and ask 'why' it is what you think it is. Challenge yourself to find features that are unequivocally associated with a cat to the point where you may only be happy to say it's a cat because it has sufficient individual factors that satisfy you that the subject in the picture has the 'essence of a cat' and that you can articulate that essence in a scientific way to justify this. This activity is a simplified test of turning 'what' into 'why' and is not as easy as you first think. Critically analysing each factor and finding out that most of the identifiable features could actually make this a dog or a goat should make you think more about other things you think are true!

This will be useful later in the chapter, I promise!

The rest of this chapter will focus on raising the profile of critical thinking and *analytical processes as an intrinsic part of your decision-making* **acumen**, *using* a range of methods as your practice develops, and which can greatly assist your practice.

By understanding the basic concepts of critical thinking, you will be able to think with more clarity, be more observant and learn to exploit more information. You will become sufficiently skilled to be able to build arguments which will form your dynamic responses to challenges, or to form hypotheses in more complex situations.

Building an argument with yourself to prove what you think you are seeing or experiencing is key to moving towards a more robust processing model, along with other stratagems such as **collaborative decision making** with colleagues and **shared decision making** with patients. Earlier chapters in this book look at **hypothetico-deduction** (as well as other decision-making models and methodologies) as appropriate models for decision making in paramedic practice, all of which require strong critical thinking skills when developing **hypotheses.**

Hypothesis generation, like many other tools and methods, requires a process too. This is where critical thinking has a strong place in your arsenal. Many situations are linked with apparently unequivocal answers – self-evident circumstances, situations or pathologies (equivalent to identifying a cat) – and it's these situations where dynamic analysis can be rapidly used to ensure a healthy level of distrust and scepticism in a positive way to ensure what you are seeing, hearing or experiencing is true. For example, think of times when you have had to cross a road that is usually busy, but now it has no traffic flowing because of an incident. The presence of an empty road suggests it's safe to cross. All you have done is identify the 'what', *the empty road* with no apparent dangers. By *not* trusting your instinct, you quickly ask *why* it is safe and consider that the expected conditions may have been altered, such as the risk/potential for other emergency vehicles travelling on the wrong side of the road to access the scene, along with the increasing risk of electric vehicles travelling much more quietly than fossil fuel powered vehicles. In clinical practice, you may be influenced by the setting you are in; for example, what would your perception of patients' disease severity be if they are able to walk onto a medivac aircraft?

This is not a deductive process *per se*; rather it's a dynamic inductive process which requires critical thinking to ensure that the reasons to act are quickly assessed rather than viewed as the truth – 'Before I act, can I trust my instinct?' In many situations, making sense of a situation must happen before actual decisions are made, and critical thinking can be considered as one of the methods of making sense of what you see. Many texts include decision making as merely an aspect of critical thinking, and this is true, but only in the dynamic sense. Arguably, in clinical practice, critical thinking crosscuts decision making and has a utility in many stages of information processing, categorization and diagnosis (or action). Put simply, critically appraise what you see, balanced alongside the other pieces of information you have; act upon it quickly when you need to and use it to shape hypotheses when more consideration is needed.

It's easy to have the intention to think critically, but making critical thinking part of your everyday processes needs attention and purposeful practice otherwise you may let your guard down, and this will affect your ability to make good judgements in values-based decision making.

Information Processing

Diagnosis is one of the cornerstones of the technical aspect of clinical practice. It provides patients with clarity about their symptoms, disease trajectory and recovery in the most holistic way possible at the time (for example, how it might affect their lifestyle, job or family). Reaching a diagnosis in practice is little more than an exercise in categorization – recognizing or comparing something against a known control. This section looks at decision making based on information processing, utilizing cycles of hypothesis and deduction in an iterative way, building and testing hypotheses, which relies upon good data being considered (critically considered and well processed). Information is usually gained from a range of sources (for instance, the patient's long-term history, their onset of illness, and other information such as physiological markers like blood pressure).

The concept of the Information Processing Model, which examines the way decision makers rationally identify and test theories and hypotheses, is very much associated with the model employed by medicine. It has begun to emerge as the systematic methodology used by paramedics to ensure that the correct decisions are made. It also contributes to developing treatment plans and referral or discharge decisions. Being able to find information and process it effectively provides the clues within the dilemmas we face in practice. These, in turn, become hypotheses needed to help solve the problem. This is a vitally important aspect of the decision-making skill of clinicians.

Remember the basic four-stage deductive process (cue acquisition, hypothesis generation, interpretation and hypothesis testing/retesting) as outlined in Elstein's hypothetico-deductive model (see p. 67). This deductive process, foundational in clinical reasoning, was further explored by Carnevali (1984), Radwin (1990) and Hamers et al. (1994). Radwin and Hamers' work built upon the principles elucidated by Elstein, providing additional insights and perspectives within a healthcare context, and created a more accessible and simplified version of the more detailed seven-stage process described by Carnevali in 1984. Both models effectively demonstrate the steps that decision makers must take to accurately reach the correct answer.

Of course, these theories assume that the information being considered is correct in the first place. The father of the computer, Charles Babbage (b. 1791, d. 1871), was once asked:

> *Pray, Mr. Babbage, if you put into the machine wrong figures, will the right answers come out?*
>
> (Babbage, 1864).

His response to the question was far from polite by all accounts. He hadn't considered that anyone would put in the wrong information, or perhaps that his machine was not capable of correcting these errors. Either way, the fact remains that if you put the wrong information in, the wrong answer is almost inevitable. In the last chapter, we looked at human factors and how the subject emerged from the experiences and adverse incidents from the aviation industry. Think back to the World Health Organization's (WHO) surgical checklist and how this prevented significant errors by 30% (p. 82). Much of the essence of the checklist is the need to sense check (process) the information before using it. For example, asking the patient which leg they are expecting to wake up with has prevented mistaken amputations. By way of contrast, in the aviation industry a notable negative event where information was incorrectly processed was the Kegworth Air Crash in January 1989. The aircraft suffered an engine fire in one engine, and because the pilot could smell smoke through the air conditioning, he assumed he could shut down the engine which runs the air-conditioning. If he had checked, he would have realized that, on the 400 series Boeing 737, the air-conditioning is run from the opposite engine to the one it is run from in the 300 series with which he was very familiar. He shut down the good engine by mistake, and then failed to understand why this action didn't resolve the problem – ultimately leading to the crash and the loss of 47 lives. The loss of one engine on a modern airliner is an inconvenience rather than a disaster, but poor information processing and making assumptions led to a disaster.

In the computing industry, poor information processing has evolved into the modern acronym of 'GIGO' – garbage in, garbage out. This has lots of applications in health decision making (and aviation). If we accept the earlier statement that deduction is no more than categorization or computation, the risk of inputting the wrong information and expecting the correct answer to come out must arguably be the greatest pitfall of the decision maker. It also has strong links with the decision to trust your old brain or your new brain (System 1/System 2) and allowing intuition to drive you (which engine will you shut down if you don't think about it?). Looking back to where we considered the use of intuition as a useful tool in creating ideas, we should be mindful that creating hypotheses is a psychological necessity. There is nothing worse than staring at something with no idea what to do. This doesn't occur where you achieve an initial intuitive feeling, as this provides reassurance and a base upon which to build the decision-making case – but it isn't the way to find the final answer. Information processing, like all aspects of decision making, is an active process and the processing is simply an assessment of probability, based on evidence or experience. (For example, if you have Professor Plum in your hand of cards when playing Cluedo, he isn't the murderer.) The information you select as ideas or hypotheses must themselves be validated to avoid correct processing of incorrect data.

The default approach, particularly in diagnostic reasoning, involves deductive reasoning rather than reliance on pure intuition. As previously discussed, however, this must not be at the expense of decisiveness in an emergency. It is important to recognize the utility of intuition when discussing hypothetico-deduction, as the information upon which deduction is based is usually derived from intuitive, experiential, or (in the worst-case scenario) tacit knowledge. Healthcare decision making often requires significant evidence of knowledge and competency – particularly in relation to the knowledge of health, disease and therapy. Clinicians, therefore, need confidence as well as competence in order to operate effectively and safely. The development of the decision-making skills is no different to learning about the diseases or treatments faced in practice.

Consider your information processing in the following scenario.

Case Example: Elliott

You are called to a 17-year-old female with abdominal pain. She is in her room accompanied by her mother. She complains of diffuse abdominal discomfort and nausea. She is usually fit and well and has an active social life.

You immediately start to draw on your knowledge (and experience, in this case) to consider some of the possible common conditions.

- Appendicitis
- Gastroenteritis
- Pregnancy
- Renal colic
- Pelvic inflammatory disease.

You ask questions relevant to each of these:

- 'Do you have your appendix?' The patient had her appendix out as a child, so this can't be appendicitis.
- 'Any diarrhoea or vomiting, and has anyone else been ill in the family?' She has no diarrhoea or vomiting, just slight nausea for two days, so it's not likely to be gastroenteritis either.

- 'Could you be pregnant?' Elliott's mother says unequivocally that she could not be, and why have you asked. (Interesting . . .)
- 'Could I test your urine please?' The patient asks if that includes a pregnancy test (Also interesting . . .)

The urine test shows that Elliott is pregnant. You are worried that her pain is a complication of early pregnancy and explain gently that you need to send her to hospital.

In this scenario, the data acquisition and processing phase elicits many statements upon which the initial hypothesis was formed. There are, however, confounding factors, which would have had a negative impact had this been overlooked. Decision makers should remain open minded and be prepared to step back when processing information in dynamic and high-pressure environments, or when they are still developing their own experience in a particular area of practice. This is different from the perception of those who have been in practice for a shorter period. The evidence shows that where clinicians lack experience, their practice is no less safe, but decisions may not be made as rapidly (Benner, 1984). This is due to the time needed to process data, create and test hypotheses.

In the scenario, the denial of sexual activity may have closed the line of questioning and examination leading to the actual diagnosis. It could have given rise to a false conclusion, supporting the deductive process of decision making. This illustrates the point that decisions should be based on sound, validated information – *garbage in, garbage out*. We assume that the patient tells the truth, even when they do not (this, of course, may be their own truth as disclosed when giving their health history) and therefore **positivism** in context to aspects such as moral judgements in history taking may lead to false information being given (denial of sexual activity leading to exclusion of obstetric causes of abdominal pain). Health professionals should perhaps avoid being cynical in front of patients, but should be open-minded and take a **post-positivist** (objective assessment of fact/truth) approach, particularly when taking a patient's history, For example, comparing the objective nature of a patient's condition with how the patient expresses it in domains such as disability or pain.

Often the initial hypothesis may be the strongest or most obvious and become the final diagnosis. It is therefore important to remember not to fall back on judgement based on its outcome and its use of intuition, as this puts us back to be driven by 'what', rather than 'why'. In the case given, the strong, most obvious hypothesis was generated intuitively based on the clinical presentation, age and gender of the patient. That embedded heuristic information had to be processed to avoid placing unwarranted faith in what appeared obvious (do we always know what we don't know?). Consider what may have happened if the patient's mother's denial, and the patient's own lack of opposition to this had been accepted at face value. Potentially, this lack of information processing and selection of a reasonable hypothesis to test could have been life threatening. Decision making is a dynamic process, based on making choices and judgements. Deliberation – careful consideration of each step taken prior to arriving at a decision or a diagnosis – is important if the patient's best interests are to be secured.

Barriers to Critical Thinking

Critical thinking is about considering how you think. It must be practised, like any task that becomes a skill. Critical thinking is a learned ability; few people have these skills innately, suggesting that practice will improve your fluency in this ability and increase its usefulness. In this way, the initial clumsiness you may experience will diminish with time. All new skills feel alien and difficult, but that shouldn't stop you from persevering. In *Bounce*, the author Matthew Syed (2011) discusses being able to become an expert following 10,000 hours of 'purposeful practice' resulting from repeated application, leading to the development of muscle memory, heuristic shortcuts, comfort and reduced cognitive load. If you are learning to play table tennis or the guitar, you may be fortunate to find a few hours each week to practise, but decades of dedication will be necessary if you are to achieve expertise. Critical thinking, however, can be practised in virtually every waking moment, and certainly during the working week. Someone practising table tennis for 40 hours each week would take just over five years to achieve 10,000 hours of practice to become an expert table tennis player, but in critical thinking if you applied your craft to every waking hour, you would achieve this in less than two years. Clearly, this is not a directly applicable analogy but serves to highlight how most endeavours take time to bed-in and become established in line with the models used in healthcare practice.

Clearly, the idea of highlighting periods of defined, purposeful practice is an exaggeration and, in reality, once you have moved on from the initial clumsy period associated with any new skill, you will not consciously switch the process on and off. In due course, you may not be aware of it to the level where you could retrospectively identify each time you thought critically. It is, however, important that you always know you are *able* to think critically so you can become conscious of where you may not be thinking critically. As this awareness diminishes, you will need to retain an awareness of where you may be prone to not thinking critically, and there are plenty of barriers to practising and using critical thinking. It is important therefore to identify these threats so you can recognize when these extrinsic factors are interfering with your practice. Before reading on, let's do a quick exercise.

Critical Thinking Exercise: Making Links and Association Bias

Read the following nursery rhyme:

Humpty Dumpty

Humpty Dumpty sat on a wall,
Humpty Dumpty had a great fall.
All the King's horses and all the King's men
Couldn't put Humpty together again.

And the following recipe:

The Ultimate Meringue

4 large organic egg whites, at room temperature

115 g caster sugar

115 g icing sugar

What immediately springs to mind as connecting these two quite disparate things – a nursery rhyme and a recipe?

The obvious answer is of course *eggs*, and why wouldn't you make that link – unless of course you were thinking critically. Perhaps go back and read the two passages again and look more carefully at what you are reading, and challenge your instinctive, intuitive response. Park your preconceptions and answer the questions '*What is the link?*' and '*Is there a link, and if so, why?*' The answer is that there is no actual evidential link whatsoever. There is nothing to state that Humpty Dumpty was an egg, and the origin of the nursery rhyme suggests no clear intent for the subject to be thought of as an egg (Hunt, 2004). We are all aware of the nursery rhyme, and the image of Humpty Dumpty as an egg has been etched into our consciousness to a point where the absence of the word 'egg' has become entirely detached from our belief that Humpty Dumpty was, in fact, an egg. Moreover, it's hard to imagine anything other than an egg when you hear the words Humpty Dumpty. In clinical care we must look for the red flags or other critical factors until we can prove there aren't any, and seek to challenge any biases or preconceived or embedded notions that could be wrong.

In yet another (albeit ground-based) aviation analogy, airport security staff looking at bags passing through the x-ray scanner do not glance at each image and assume there is nothing sinister, they ask the vital question every time a bag passes – and it's the same question you must ask yourself: '*Where is the bomb?*' (Rosenorn-Lanng, 2014, p. 1).

It is also worth noting for completeness that there is a vegan recipe for meringue, which uses chickpea brine – aquafaba – instead of egg whites. Where more information is available, linking Humpty Dumpty and meringue may elicit no evidence of eggs at all!

Now we have worked through a very specific exercise where we may have been betrayed by a longstanding childhood belief, let's look at some other barriers to critical thinking. The contents in the following table are arguably the cornerstones of the barriers to critical thinking and were developed by Dr Richard Paul and Dr Linda Elder from the Foundation for Critical Thinking (Paul & Elder, 2001). These five headings resonate with healthcare practice and support the argument that we as humans are flawed thinkers due to competing personality traits, influences, biases and fallacies. Remember, if you cannot think critically, you cannot develop hypotheses, which are essential to the more complex decision-making processes covered later in the book.

Table 5.1 is taken from *The Miniature Guide to Critical Thinking: Concepts and Tools* by Paul and Elder (2001).

Table 5.1 Breaking Down Critical Thinking

Concept	Definition	Impact
'It's true because I believe it.'	**Innate egocentrism** I assume that what I believe is true even though I have never questioned the basis for many of my beliefs. ***Example:*** *'You can never give a patient too much oxygen.'*	Harm to the patient
'It's true because we believe it.'	**Innate sociocentrism** I assume that the dominant beliefs of the groups to which I belong are true even though I have never questioned the basis for those beliefs. ***Example:*** *'We have always done it this way at my ambulance station.' (Tribal behaviour)*	Development of toxic cultures, unwarranted variation and poor outcomes for patients.
'It's true because I want to believe it.'	**Innate wish fulfilment** I believe what 'feels good', what does not require me to change my thinking in any significant way, and what does not require me to admit I have been wrong. ***Example:*** *'It's fine to stay with every patient as long as I like. I don't believe it affects other patients or my colleagues.'*	Behaviour or thinking is embedded based on prior feelings without reflection or insight being sought.
'It's true because I have always believed it.'	**Innate self-validation** I have a strong desire to maintain beliefs I have long held, even though I have not seriously considered the extent to which those beliefs are justified by the evidence. ***Example:*** *'I was shown this method on my technician course 20 years ago – why should I do it differently now?'*	Failure to explore new ways of thinking or working, and which lead to dogged or entrenched views or behaviours.

(continued)

Table 5.1 Breaking Down Critical Thinking (*Continued*)

Concept	Definition	Impact
'It's true because it is in my interest to believe it.'	**Innate selfishness** I believe whatever justifies my getting more power, or personal advantage even though those beliefs are not grounded in sound reasoning or evidence. ***Example:*** *'I don't believe that any patient wouldn't want to be resuscitated, so I carry out advanced life support on every patient regardless. It's my professional registration at stake after all!'*	Misplaced feeling of needing to act with self-preservation based on what felt safe in the past.

Egotism *vs* Humility

We all like to believe that we are competent, and that our knowledge and skills are of a high standard. It is important – perhaps even vital – to park any preconceptions you may have (or may develop) about a situation due to your position within the care team, such as rank or seniority. There are many examples of where ego or a lack of insight leads to poor interpersonal relationships, and cause harm. While more and more clinical encounters managed by paramedics happen outside of the traditional ambulance crew configuration, critical thinking can and should occur within any relationship during an encounter (professional/carer, professional/family, professional/professional etc.), and perhaps the most important relationship to work on is between you and your ego. Building an argument with yourself is a crucial skill, and much harder in many ways than being challenged by a colleague.

Much of the work to improve safety in aviation has its origins in engineering the conditions humans work in as a method of reducing human error and recognizing human flaws and limitations (such as ego and hierarchy). These approaches are key aspects of what are known as **human factors** (Rutherford, 2020), and consider the need to design work around the aspects of human nature that can influence decisions and outcomes (Rosenorn-Lanng, 2014). The Tenerife air disaster, which occurred on 27 March 1977, typifies a situation where a lack of insight (and ego) displayed by the pilot of the KLM Boeing 747, and the fear shown by the first officer who chose not to challenge his pilot's decision (despite strongly believing that something was wrong), led to the deaths of over 500 people on the runway that day. As with most large-scale accidents, there are wider factors than simply the interactions of human beings, as described by Sydney Dekker in his book *Drift into Failure* (Dekker, 2011). The following passage is taken from the Spanish Authority's investigation report:

> ***5.2. Authority in the Cockpit.*** *Although nothing abnormal can be deduced from the CVR (Cockpit Voice Recorder), the fact exists that a co-pilot not very experienced with [Boeing] 747s was flying with one of the pilots of greatest prestige in the company who was, moreover, KLM's chief flying instructor and*

> *who had certified him fit to be a crew member for this type of aeroplane. In case of doubt, these circumstances could have induced the co-pilot not to ask any questions and to assume that this captain was always right.*
>
> Aviation Safety Network, n.d.

Today, any member of flight crew can challenge the captain, as the development of 'graded assertiveness' (Madden, 2018) helped to flatten hierarchies and improve communication. This approach has, with varying success, transferred to parts of healthcare. In the operating theatre setting, for example, any clinician or other team member – doctor, nurse, operating department practitioner, porter – is encouraged to speak out where they perceive a problem, using structured briefings throughout the perioperative pathway as described in the WHO Surgical Checklist (Sign In, Time Out, Sign Out) (World Health Organization, 2009). This has led to the avoidance of serious errors, such as the removal of incorrect limbs or organs, but challenges do exist with consistency and distractions (HSIB, 2021b).

The journey to becoming a good decision maker and critical thinker involves understanding our own limitations in terms of how we perceive ourselves. This itself requires the emergence of humility over ego, and an assessment of our own true belief in our own abilities. We tend to overstate our abilities (see Chapter 4 – the Dunning-Kruger Effect – Dunning and Kruger, 1999). This can lead to our ego or **sociocentricity** (akin to groupthink) to diminish our objectivity. You can use concepts such as the Dreyfus Model, used by Benner (1984) in *From Novice to Expert*, to assist with your own introspection and build on the balance between ego and humility. In simple terms, the more of a novice you are, the more humility you should display. It is fine to accept that you don't know something rather than to guess and cause your patient harm (see Figure 5.2).

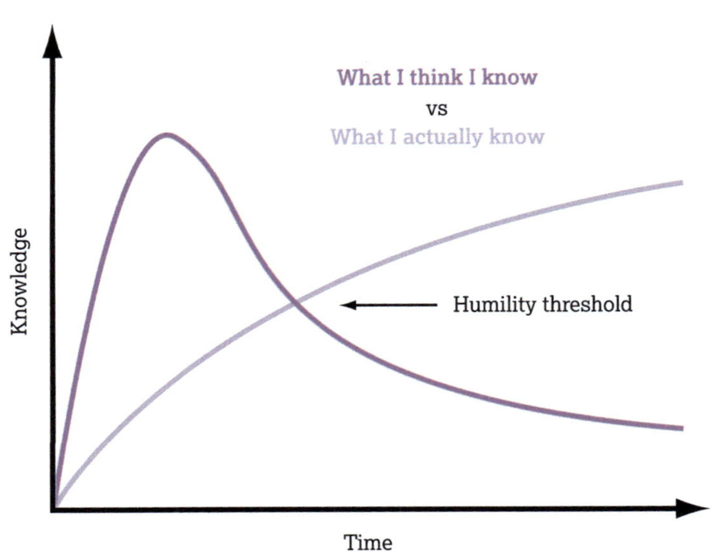

Figure 5.2 Mount Stupid – Knowledge vs Experience.

Source: Graphic adapted from Joseph F. Paris Jr., Available online: https://josephparis.me/my-articles/lessons-from-mt-stupid/.

Selfishness: Emotional Influence and Personal Values

Clinicians must make decisions with patients and respect their views, beliefs and wishes. It is not uncommon to come across a patient who has full **mental capacity** but makes an apparently bad decision about their own care. Thinking back to the beliefs we hold, and how we develop these beliefs, you may find it distressing for someone to decide that they do not wish for their treatable condition to be cured because you may have been brought up in a particular way or have developed strong views throughout life – perhaps in response to a similar life event.

Emotional drivers and values are personal to the individual, and we cannot make good decisions that are contrary to the patient's wishes, however outwardly unwise these may be, as these are a core principle of patient choice and humans' right to self-determination. You may find yourself concerned that if you agree a plan of care that supports a patient to die at home, their relatives will complain, and this will lead to disciplinary action. The experience of feeling these fears and other emotions is very real and can cloud one's judgement. Therefore, it is important to learn to understand how to suspend your own beliefs in order to uphold the patient's wishes, and how this can lead to the decision made being correct rather than imposed based on your values, and therefore wrong.

Other Important Barriers to Critical Thinking

If you search the internet or academic sources using the term 'barriers to critical thinking', you will be able to find almost every aspect of human consciousness and personality trait that can get in the way of critiquing what you see. There are many academic texts that focus on specific areas, such as building arguments, challenging experts and negotiating, but in the context of healthcare decision making, focus should be on those factors that actively or passively promote doing the best for the patient, rather than perhaps the more esoteric concepts.

Table 5.2 can be used to explore the more specific barriers to critical thinking and uses examples linked to healthcare practice. When you review these terms, you may recognize some of the traits in yourself and others, and this can be alarming. Healthcare professionals may view themselves as entirely rational and intelligent beings. The thought that superstition or wishful thinking could enter a health encounter is somewhat alien, but these two examples are seen often in hospitals. Many nurses will open the window in a room where a patient has died – a superstition. Our innate desire for our patients to have a good outcome is often wishful thinking, but we do it anyway. These are fairly harmless barriers to critical thinking, but where concepts like pride, denial and infallibility are introduced, these present very real threats to patients and must be better understood.

Table 5.2 Barriers to Critical Thinking

Barrier	Example
Absolutism	This barrier assumes that there are no exceptions, and that rules or tenets are absolute. Some ethical considerations are absolutist and may link to concepts such as human rights. Where appropriate, this is a positive concept, but in healthcare it may be too constrained and lead to poor decisions being made – particularly where they are based on an incorrect belief (e.g., taking every patient to hospital to avoid ever getting a complaint).
An over-reliance on feelings	Intuition is an example of over-reliance on feelings, and is often considered as 'gut feelings', or actions resulting from emotional influence rather than scientific or deductive enquiry.
Cognitive dissonance	Conflict or inconsistency in thoughts and beliefs. In healthcare, an example could be in the context of Making Every Contact Count (MECC) and encouraging a patient to stop smoking while still being a smoker yourself.
Conformism	This is most commonly a manifestation displayed where guidelines are applied in a rote way and used as rules that are applied to the letter and to the exclusion of other considerations.
Debilitating fear and uncertainty	In the paramedic practice setting, this barrier is associated with fear of being disciplined at work or being struck off by the regulator. Conversely, this fear may create worse decisions and provide inferior care for the patient; it is similar to the absolutist approach, taking every patient to hospital in order to avoid criticism, thus failing to make proper decisions.
Denial	This may be one of the more troubling barriers to critical thinking, and in our practice settings may be experienced in situations where a procedure has been carried out to a poor standard, but the clinician convinces him or herself that it is fine – perhaps a cannula that won't flush, which should be removed and another attempt made.
Disturbing one's comfort	Allowing ourselves to operate in the 'comfort zone' may lead to a lack of challenge, reflection and insight. Our comfort should be disturbed in order to think critically and avoid a stagnated approach.

(*continued*)

Table 5.2 Barriers to Critical Thinking (*Continued*)

Barrier	Example
Fear of being wrong or face-saving	Who wants to be wrong? One of the main demonstrable traits of an active learner and critical thinker is the lack of fear of being wrong and working collaboratively to ensure the correct outcome. Some people will not try in order to avoid failing (for instance, never taking a driving test in case you fail).
Fear of change or an unwillingness to change	We have discussed several times throughout this book the changing face of healthcare and the constantly changing patient profiles and behaviours.
Lack of discernment	Discernment is at the heart of critical thinking – considering and deciding on the quality or veracity of evidence or arguments. If you avoid discernment, you are not a critical thinker.
Lack of humility	Linked very closely to egocentrism, a lack of humility (often manifested as arrogance or overplaying experience) leads to poorly structured decision making and intuitive judgements. Humility is a trait associated with confident people with smaller egos, who reflect on their practice.
Narrow-mindedness or close-mindedness	How often have we heard a colleague say they don't believe in something? In healthcare, the evidence base changes often and we must keep pace. Fixing on concepts that become outmoded is an example of where narrow-mindedness can impede critical thinking.
Peer-pressure	If you subscribe to the notion that there are no bad apples, only bad barrels, the influence of peer-pressure could exist in a positive or negative way. Peer-pressure implies conformity to an established norm or a culture that prevents challenge. Remember that history tells us following orders is no defence. Neither is citing peer-pressure.
Pride	A dent in your pride is rarely fatal, so don't approach practice with the intention of preserving it at all costs. Being wrong is important and allows reflection and learning. It's better to experience a loss of pride than have to explain to a coroner why you acted as you did.
Sociocentrism or **ethnocentrism**	In the same way we associate peer-pressure as a barrier to critical thinking, groupthink and cultural beliefs to which you subscribe (or are expected to subscribe) also diminish effective reasoning.

(*continued*)

Table 5.2 Barriers to Critical Thinking (*Continued*)

Barrier	Example
Stereotyping	This is much rarer now due to the work undertaken across health and social care to recognise diversity and vulnerabilities. On occasion though, some patients are unfairly grouped and stereotyped based on factors which are not directly relevant (see Chapter 3). For instance, frequent callers/attenders may be dismissed as a nuisance, leading to their issues not being resolved. Critically appraising why patients return time and again will promote the correct decision for their onward care.
Wishful thinking	'I am sure this will be fine'. You aren't sure, and this is not a good basis for resolving an episode of patient care. Remember that most errors and poor judgements don't cause harm and go undetected. One of the core tenets of this book is to remove doubt and avoid wishful thinking.

Intuition and Experience in Critical Thinking

There is a theme throughout this book which suggests that intuition is a bad thing if not closely monitored, and that experience is only as good as the time spent reflecting and consolidating it after the event. What this does *not* mean is that the acquisition of experiences should not lead to faster access to problem solving in parallel with progressing towards expertise, particularly when you are using inductive reasoning. Intuition should always be critically appraised where time permits whenever a similar situation occurs (such as the approach to the patient in cardiac arrest, where protocol determines action and action is informed by situational awareness). Where you clearly know what should be done in a given situation, that shouldn't stop you acting where it is very obvious. But where decisions are difficult to reach, some level of critical thinking must occur, even if this does not progress to a full processing of the situation (using hypothetico-deduction).

Figure 5.3 shows a useful way of adopting a method of thinking critically in high-pressure situations requiring action. Take a moment to walk through the flowchart using different scenarios you have faced in practice and see which route you take. The first junction in the flowchart, which assesses the typicality of the situation, is a very useful prompt and allows a rapid use of experience and intuition based on a repeatable process, which takes almost no time at all.

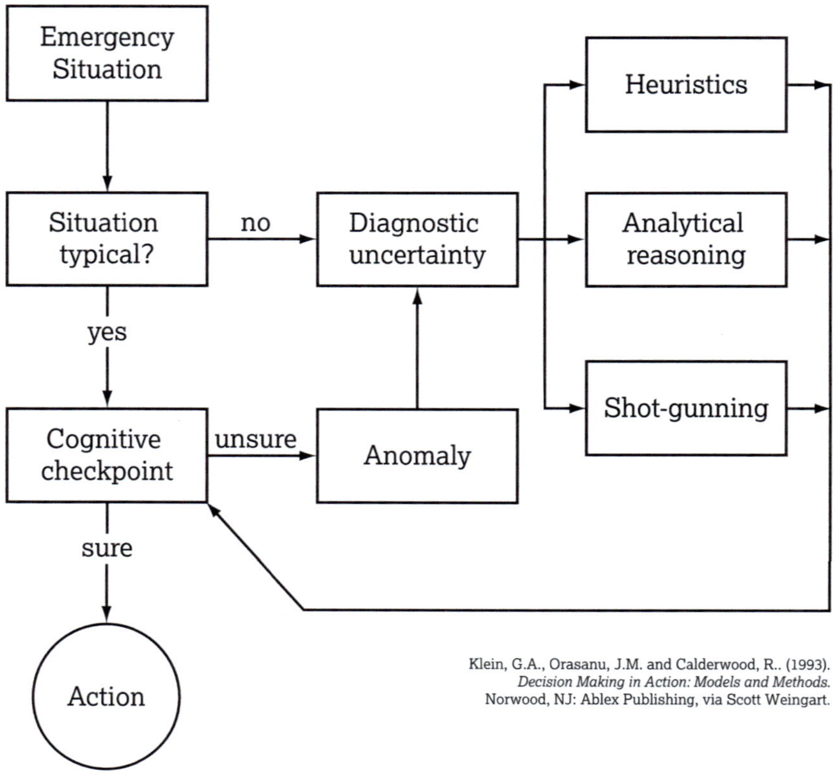

Figure 5.3 Decision making in action: models and methods.
Source: Klein et al., 1993

Decision Point Management: Taking Control at Each Stage

There is a game you may have heard of called bagatelle. It is similar to pinball in that a small ball is sent up to the top of a runway and then falls down towards a series of numbered holes at the bottom. These decrease in value from the centre out to the ones at the edge. Between the holes and the top of the runway are pins, which are intended to deflect the ball randomly, meaning there is no more skill involved in achieving a higher score than a lower score; however, the ball is far more likely to land in one of the lower scored holes, as the pins tend to move the ball away from the centre line. Unlike pinball, there are no flippers to send the ball back up the runway, and other than the speed at which the ball is sent up to the top of the runway, the player's ability to influence the outcome is minimal. This is a useful way to describe the use of decision point management as an alternative to random acts. Each pin that can randomly deflect you represents the small decisions you make, which make up the overall outcome – such as in a diagnostic process. Decision point management requires each pin to become a considered judgement, rather than a random act, and for each level to be navigated as an active process, rather than just letting fate take its course. The correct answer is the result of navigating these multiple forks in the road.

If your game of Bagatelle has eighteen rows of pins offset with the pins below, and each column has eight or nine pins (see Figure 5.4), would you be able to recall

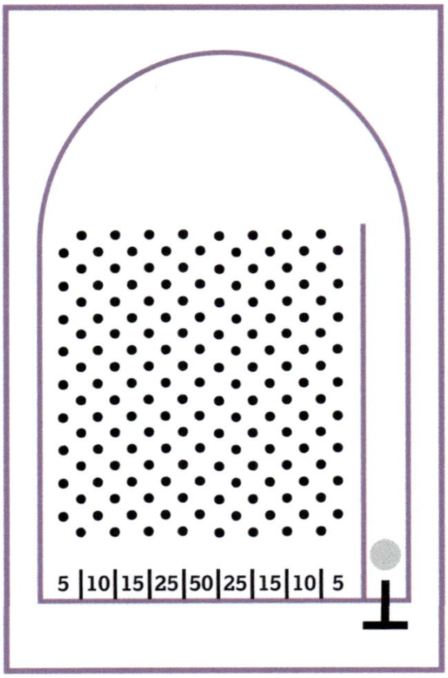

Figure 5.4 Bagatelle 1.

exactly which pins your ball hit on its way down the board? Were your intentions to get a high score met?

While not a decision-making strategy in itself, decision point management is an important tool to use when reviewing and reflecting on the overall outcome, diagnosis or decision. At each point did you know where you were in the process? Did you know the likely outcomes based on each pin hit? Did you think forward as events progressed? Can you look back to see where you should have changed direction? While bagatelle is essentially a random undertaking at the point you launch the ball, by the time it hits the first pin you can start to consider the critical path, albeit in slow time. In much the same way, by noting the level at which an infarct occurs in the coronary circulation and how much collateral circulation the patient has, it is possible to envision the limitations of which regions of the heart will be affected, and to what degree. In real terms, you can simplify the game by removing pins at each level, localizing the possible path for the ball each time it reaches the next level of pins (Figure 5.5).

Once the ball falls between two pins on the top row, the other pins are out of play and so on down the board at each level.

Figure 5.6 shows the bagatelle board a few levels later. The shaded area is larger still leaving areas of the playing surface that are now inaccessible.

Figure 5.7 depicts the last level. There are only two possible routes left. In healthcare, these are your final differential diagnoses or impressions. Because you tracked the route through the game, rather than making it random, you can better control the outcome, critically appraising each fork in the road.

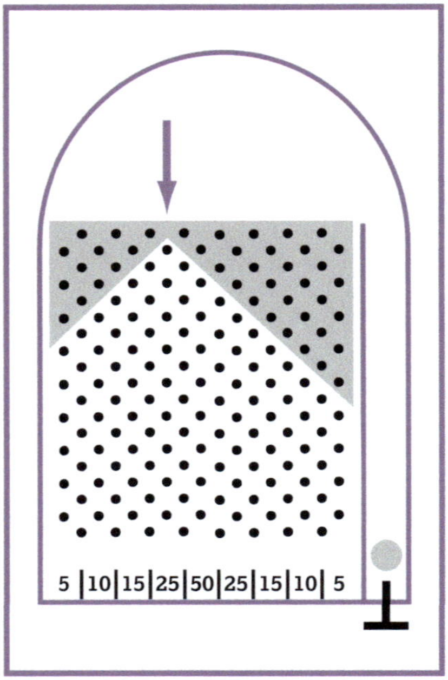

Figure 5.5 Bagatelle 2.

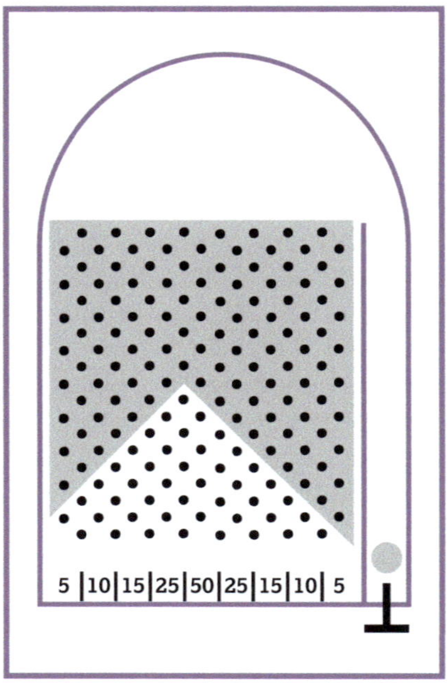

Figure 5.6 Bagatelle 3.

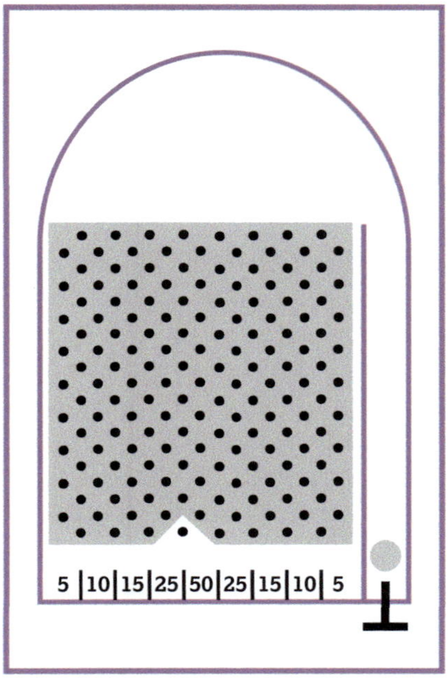

Figure 5.7 Bagatelle 4.

When thinking critically, imagine where you are on the board and how much of it is irrelevant based on what part of the board cannot be accessed – critically considering what is clearly out of scope (e.g., ignoring pregnancy-related issues for male patients). If further down the board you realize that information in another part of the board is needed, this indicates that you made errors further up the board.

As you get better at critical thinking and have removed the barriers that impede the way to make small conclusions along the way, you will find yourself needing to back-track less. Imagine that the information needed to find the answer to the Humpty Dumpty exercise is higher up the board, and that the critical thinking applied allowed transition through that part of the board. The final piece of the puzzle therefore is entering the board at the correct point to minimize the random nature by which you move down the bagatelle board. Suddenly you have gone from riding the bagatelle board as a passenger, to controlling where the ball enters the game and steering each contact with the pins to ensure the route is better controlled. Should you need to go back, you know where the incorrect deviation was made.

Clearly this analogy lacks some of the real-world traits that we see in clinical practice, and the two-dimensional description doesn't lend itself well to the realities of the complex cues, hints and information sources with which we are bombarded, not to mention the constellational, interdependent and interrelational reality of patient care. The point about the barriers to critical thinking being ever present and sending you down cognitive blind alleys is illustrated in this method, and as we move ahead you can see how a real-world example is about converting what may feel like a random or self-determining event into a controlled and cognitively derived event. Imagine if the ball represented chest pain as the patient's major symptom group, and instead of scores there were diagnoses across the bottom of the board. How comfortable would you be allowing the diagnosis of indigestion to be made?

Summing Up: Moving from 'What' to 'Why'

The first step towards better hypothetico-deductive decision making relies on clean data – information that has been filtered and verified before use as a preparatory stage in the decision-making process. It isn't enough to simply say what you see, and being able to satisfy yourself as to why something is the way it is will assist greatly when higher level decisions are made; this, in turn, will ensure your patients are as safe as possible and allow you to consolidate each experience you have without needing to accept each individual episode as obvious or, worse, always correct in hindsight. It is true that with the vast majority of encounters with patients and their pathologies, it will be blindingly obvious what is wrong, but these situations always have a backstory, and it is the acceptance, or otherwise, of what you see that will help you grow as a decision-maker and a critical thinker. Establishing the balance between System-1 and System-2 thinking in the context of critical thinking is hard to achieve, and your reliance on each system will develop over time.

By way of example, experienced clinicians may commence cardiopulmonary resuscitation without taking a pulse. At this point the 'what' is unequivocal, and decisive/swift action becomes of paramount importance (System-1 processing). This instant access to the 'essence of pulselessness' is conceptually identical to the 'essence of cat' (p. 117–118) in that the context, situation, signs, features and other subtle indications all speak loudly to the correct answer. If you are wrong, the patient will wake up and tell you to get off, and you can then consider the 'why'– why did I initially think they needed CPR? If you are right, you can start asking why they are pulseless in parallel with the essential treatment (System-2 processing).

Conclusion

This chapter has introduced the concept of critical thinking, applied in a practical way, and intended to promote its use in a way that improves one's approach to situations that appear obvious but may not always be so. It is important to make sure that each situation is approached in such a way that the rapidly emerging picture, based on a wide variety of information, is seen through sceptical and cynical eyes. This will produce the required impetus to be inquisitive and probing. As with many theories and models, the world is rarely that simple, and there will always be other dilemmas and conundrums that need to be overcome in practice.

The next chapter will start to look at the more holistic aspects of decision making, moving the theory into a more parallel position alongside patient-centred care. By the end of the book, the skills discussed will always be subordinate to the patient's needs, rather than being a superficial skill from which the clinician derives satisfaction. Rather, it is the effect this ability has on the patient outcome overall that becomes most important. As you implement critical thinking into your practice as part of your developing decision-making skills, you will need to start thinking about the other considerations to hone your art, such as improving your communication skills, ethical considerations, managing changing and dynamic environments, and considering the evidence base in the context of patients' needs and wishes.

Reflective Exercises

1. Consider a time when you have worked with a more senior clinician or have been in a situation where you have witnessed a senior–subordinate team dynamic. What risks were present? Could harm have been caused to the patient? And what techniques could you use to prevent errors caused by this type of issue in the practice setting?
2. Consider the list of issues from the section on 'Barriers to Critical Thinking'. Work through these and reflect on times when you have been affected by these barriers. Consider ways you might control this in the future and how this can support safer decision making.
3. Think about a clinical decision you have made (diagnosis, treatment or management), and try to work back to each fork in the road you managed. Did you consider concepts such as acuity assessment, patient factors or external influences? How could you make these decisions better in the future?

Further Resources

Visit the Foundation for Critical Thinking website (www.criticalthinking.org) to learn more about critical thinking.

Chapter 6

The Garden Gate Test: Putting Decision-Making Theory into Practice

Andy Collen and Si Robinson

Chapter Objectives

This chapter will cover:

- **The cognitive continuum** – how and when to use intuitive decisions in paramedic practice safely, and when to shift to deliberation when facing more complex cases
- **Experience and competence** – an exploration of the Benner model 'From Novice to Expert' and Dreyfus's 'Model of Expertise'; we consider how these can be applied in our decision making
- **Judgement and sense making** – interpreting and reflecting on decisions in order to make improved decisions in the future.

Introduction

This chapter is called 'The Garden Gate Test' and that needs an explanation. The Garden Gate Test is a way of challenging yourself, ensuring that you have confidence in your decisions and that you are confident that you have provided the best care for your patient before you or they walk away. The test originated from the experience of getting to the patient's garden gate after discharging them at home following a 911 call, and already worrying whether your decision was correct. This metaphor could be replaced with a patient leaving your consulting room, or any other paramedic practice setting. If you find yourself reaching for the gate latch (or watching the patient reaching for the door handle to leave) and are already considering the consequences if things go wrong, you have made the wrong decision – even if the decision is technically correct. Doubting yourself in this way may or may not mean that you have not made an unequivocal and defensible decision, and it's really important for your own wellbeing that you move on from each completed encounter in order to focus on caring for your next patient. This includes diagnostic decisions as well as treatment and/or management decisions, and can be part of safety netting for the patient's benefit.

Moving theory into practice can be very challenging, and the dilemmas discussed in the previous chapters all link to the concepts discussed in this chapter. These concepts will lead to new skills, which can be used in clinical encounters. As with all skills, once these have been acquired, they need to be consolidated to ensure that the approach can be used effectively when providing patient care. It is vital to promote confidence in clinical practice, and there are plenty of opportunities to create anxiety – particularly if you are making complex decisions.

This chapter will focus on understanding and using the theoretical models discussed throughout this book, developing reasoned decisions that factor knowledge and experience, the nature of the situation, and how to choose the optimal mode of decision-making in order to make a safe and effective decision. A theme running throughout the chapter is the importance of utilizing these concepts beyond clinical decisions alone, for instance, building a picture of neglect in a vulnerable person, in addition to vague situations where a definitive diagnosis (or even an impression) is unlikely. Remember too that the decision to give an intervention is the culmination of a diagnostic process and forms an important aspect of practice. As your diagnostic, therapeutic and management acumen develops, you may want to build on your fundamental deductive decision-making skills, using inductive and abductive reasoning in your practice.

Like any competency-based skill, you will be prone to making skills-based errors (slips and lapses) and mistakes (rule breaking, knowledge), as all human beings are. Cognitive skills need practice, supervision, reflection, test and challenge; all within the same professionally supportive system that you practise in. Take care not to put your patient at risk when using your new skills – seek support and guidance when needed to ensure you are practising safely.

By the end of this chapter, you will have a much better idea of how to approach decision making dilemmas in everyday practice, and you will begin to develop your decision-making skills by putting theory into practice. This will then take you on to the next chapter, which will look in detail at drawing together these separate concepts and linking them into a single process that can improve the way you make decisions and judgements, and be safer for your patients, making your role more enjoyable and less stressful.

Defining the Cognitive Continuum

The cognitive continuum theory was created by Kenneth Hammond from the University of Colorado in 1981 and has its origins in psychology rather than healthcare. The initial theory was transposed into a health perspective in the late 1980s by Robert Hamm from the University of Oklahoma. Hamm (1988) pulled together the component theories of deduction and intuition into a single process with six modes of enquiry ranging from pure science at one extreme, and pure intuition at the other (Figure 6.1). Decision making moving around the middle ground in this gradient is known as **quasi-rationality** ('quasi' = resembling and 'rationality' = with reason). Quasi-rationality is the product of the application of the cognitive continuum – eliciting the decision based on a blend of intuition and cognition – and

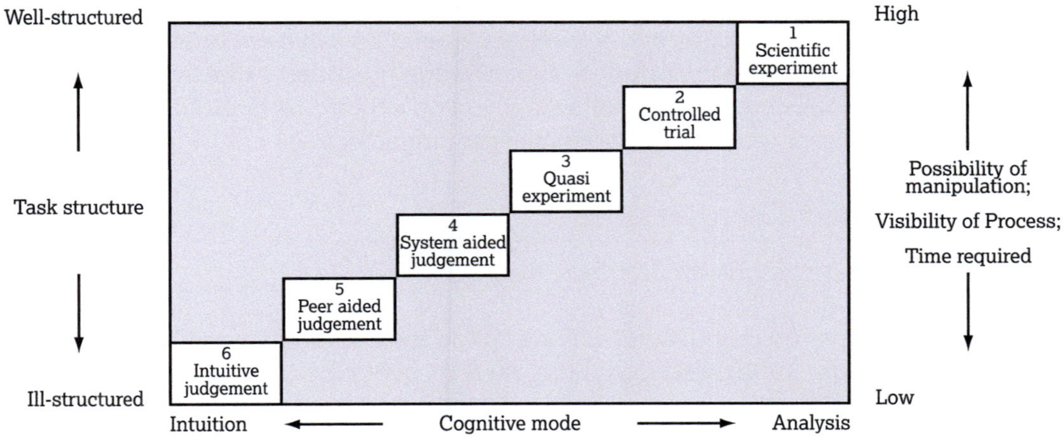

Figure 6.1 Six modes of enquiry.
Source: Hamm, 1988

requires the user to process accurate and appropriate hypotheses. The six modes of enquiry described by Hamm have clear demarcation, and yet the decision making needs to move on a sliding scale up and down the cognitive continuum. This is particularly true in the paramedic practice setting, where clinicians have access to science (such as blood tests) and absolute intuition (heuristics). Decisions can be made at the poles of cognitive continuum theory and may therefore lack either intuition or analysis. But for the most part the bounded reality of quasi-rationality provides the basis for decisions to be founded on the prevailing availability of factors, or the seeking of further evidence to refer to and test.

Many of the studies undertaken into decision-making methods suggest that clinicians in their early years of practice choose either intuition or analysis, often based on their educational background or the influence of senior colleagues and supervisors. As practice develops and experience emerges, more trust is often placed in intuition. Limited empirical support is sought, and often only achieved tacitly. As professional practice develops, we should move forward using reasoning, but we may retain a more novice approach, which does not keep pace with time in practice, and which tends to look back on experiences to achieve a decision. Experience is often regarded as a strong asset in healthcare roles. While more experienced clinicians can generate hypotheses more rapidly and easily, however, deductive ability is no more effective in the expert practitioner than the novice (if applied competently and diligently). The expert user of the cognitive continuum is able to move fluidly within it; gaining new information, testing, retesting, validating and rejecting information dynamically – demonstrating further that experience and skill in processing information can contribute to more effective decision making. When used dynamically, the cognitive continuum is like the game snakes and ladders – making progress towards a decision only to lose ground rapidly on the next roll of the dice.

That said, a criticism of the continuum is that any decision can be as simple or as complex as an individual makes it. To use the cognitive continuum effectively, the clinician must have a certain level of ability in their knowledge domain, a minimum level of competency in practice and a level of experience sufficient to confidently approach the problem. The importance of knowledge has been extensively discussed in previous chapters; the following section explores the relationship of experience and competence to confident clinical judgement.

Experience and Competence

I have been doing this job for 30 years, mate!

There is a phenomenon that afflicts humans called the Dunning-Kruger Effect (Dunning and Kruger, 1999). It suggests that novices overstate their abilities, whereas experts understate their abilities and are at increased risk due to the extent of their exposure to that risk. Both groups are at risk because of their high levels of confidence, and Figure 6.2 demonstrates this. Based on the graph, one may believe that experience is favourable, and we are going to discuss this point to ensure that experience is approached cautiously using a very non-healthcare example.
In the world of motorsports, and in particular Formula 1, Dunning-Kruger can be seen actively in talented rookies who crash less as they gain experience. A current example is Max Verstappen, the Dutch F1 driver who drives for the Red Bull team. From the moment he joined F1 from F2 it was clear that he was hugely talented, but his lack of experience in his early seasons saw him develop a reputation for

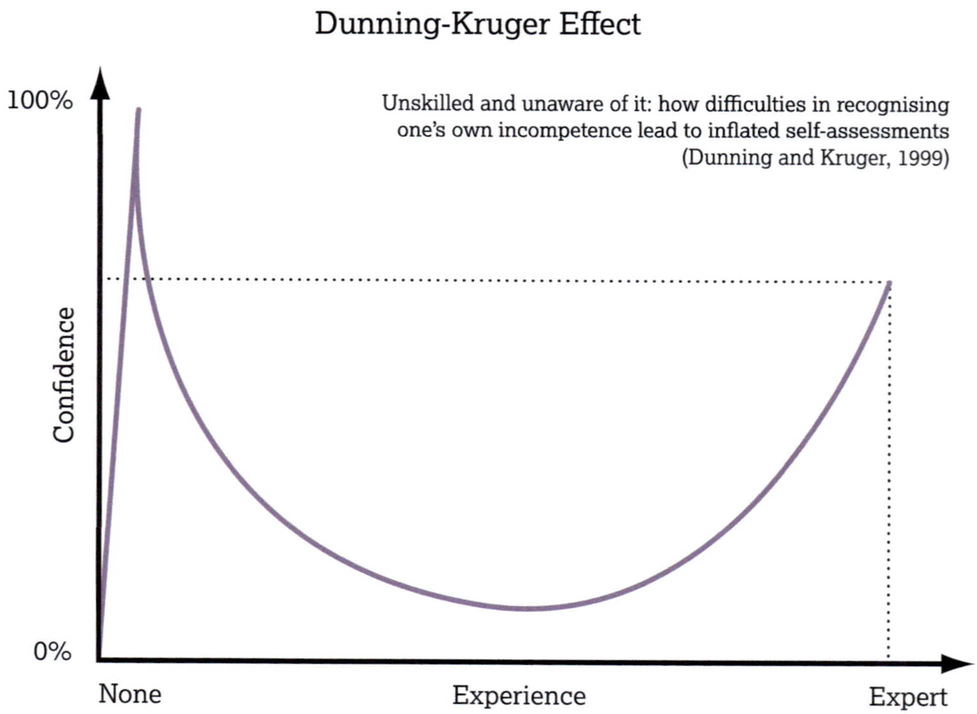

Figure 6.2 The Dunning-Kruger effect.

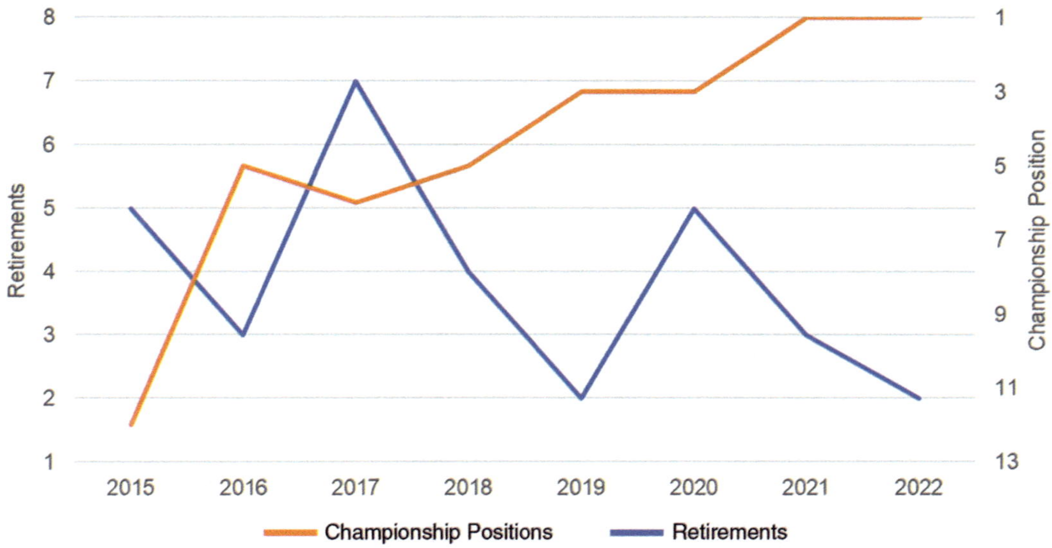

Figure 6.3 Max Verstappen's Formula 1 career statistics to 2023.
Source: https://www.statsf1.com/en/max-verstappen.aspx

being hot-headed and prone to crashing and damaging his car, which led to his 'did not finish' (DNF) rate being more than double in his early season versus his career winning seasons. In Figure 6.3 it's evident that his retirement rate and championship winning rate is not unlike the Dunning-Kruger curve if you take championship position as a proxy for confidence and the DNF rate for experience. Admittedly, not very scientific, but hopefully a helpful example to reflect on. Another point that may be pertinent is that racing drivers may also cause other drivers to DNF when collisions or other unsportsmanlike behaviours are displayed, and part of the maturity of many racing drivers is evidenced by using their consolidated experience to read the race conditions and attempt less risky overtakes, opting instead to trust the team strategy to work in their favour, such as pitstop strategies.

In paramedic practice, this can be likened to walking on scene and assessing the situation, recognizing when assistance is immediately required or when action needs to be taken, and taking a strategic, as well as tactical view, of the patient encounter. A less-experienced paramedic may be tempted to bring additional equipment (or conversely not enough) to a paediatric callout or fail to request assistance when it is most needed, thinking that the situation can be managed as a crew of two. Alternatively, the very experienced paramedic may reason that acutely unwell children tend to be non-critical (e.g., the last 100 paediatric callouts with difficulty in breathing were fine), perhaps not mentally preparing to be suddenly confronted with a rapidly deteriorating child. Experience, and importantly insight,[1] is about remaining sensitive to the Dunning-Kruger effect.

[1] Time served does not necessarily equate to increased insight unless the individual has actively reflected on their abilities as a paramedic. The importance of self-development, reflection and CPD cannot be stated enough, turning the 'what' into 'why' rather than a career of adhering to protocols and asking no questions of oneself.

This suggests therefore that there are stages of development that must be navigated and understood before experience is worth anything, and that newly acquired skills should be approached with modest self-deprecation rather than with exuberant hubris. There are seminal texts in healthcare literature that support this, and the book by Patricia Benner (*From Novice to Expert)* advocates the Dreyfus model, which describes five stages in the progression from 'novice' to 'expert' in nursing practice (Benner, 1984):

- Novice
- Advanced beginner
- Competent
- Proficient
- Expert.

How do find your place on this scale? You may be reading this book as an undergraduate paramedic student, or a postgraduate moving into specialist or advanced practice. Regardless of where you think you are on the scale above, your place between 'novice' and 'expert' is only ever commensurate with your consolidated experience and competency, and your ability to apply introspection. This means that your career may feel like a game of snakes and ladders when you reassess yourself or as you move into a new level of practice. Developing this insight should actually improve your perception of yourself as a clinician, and enhance your career by inspiring new career goals and giving you aspirations to further improve the care you offer.

Building on this, there are other notable models that use steps in a scale, and which provide opportunities to assess yourself against the Dreyfus model. The steps in Table 6.1 can be aligned to the Dreyfus model, and support the basic principle that you need to assess your competence and abilities to ensure that you use your experience alongside your knowledge and insight in order to provide more certainty that you will come up with the correct answer.

Table 6.1 Levels of Expertise

Score	Socrates/Rumsfeld*	'Maslow' (Broadwell)
1	I don't know what I don't know	Unconsciously incompetent
2	I know what I don't know	Consciously incompetent
3	I know what I know	Consciously competent
4	I don't know what I know	Unconsciously competent

This citation adapts and combines quotes by Socrates and the late Donald Rumsfeld (US Secretary of Defence, 1975–1977 and 2001–2006). Socrates defined the intellectually derived and respected 'Socratic Paradox**', and Rumsfeld made a famously rambling speech, which attempted to make a similar point.*

Linked closely to the Dreyfus model are the four stages of competence associated with Abraham Maslow, although a specific citation cannot be found in his major works, and they can most likely be attributed to Broadwell (1969). These four stages, referred to as Maslow's Hierarchy of Competence, describe very effectively the journey from novice to expert and provide a place to reflect on the pitfalls of gaps in knowledge linked to overconfident, entirely experiential and intuitive decision making without the safety net of effective deductive reasoning. They also provide a place to ensure that any **illusory superiority** is challenged.

The Four Stages of Competence

- **Unconscious incompetence** – The subject has no insight into their lack of understanding or skill. They may not place any value in the skill (for example, I don't believe in 12-lead EGC; 3-lead is fine) or be unwilling to learn, despite encouragement.
- **Conscious incompetence** – The subject has the insight sufficient to recognize they do not have understanding or skill. They may want to learn new skills and have a will to resolve the knowledge gap.
- **Conscious competence** – The subject knows they are capable of the skill and understands it. They may not find it easy and may have to concentrate intently to achieve the outcome from the skill. The execution may lack fluency and flow and appear deliberate.
- **Unconscious competence** – The subject carries out the skill to such a degree as to be 'second nature'. Some psychomotor examples may be seen as 'muscle memory', and the subject may be able to do other tasks simultaneously. The subject is competent to the level of being able to teach others.

By way of example, let's take three different paramedics and assess them for their place on the Novice to Expert scale, based on the steps in Table 6.1.

- Stacey is a newly qualified paramedic. She came top of her class and is now a registered healthcare professional. She passed the course; she gets to drive with visual and audible warning systems and put cannulae into patients; she thinks she is invincible and that she has all the accumulated knowledge and skills needed for pre-hospital care.
- Jameel is a paramedic who qualified 15 years ago. He has 'been there, done that' and is the quintessentially unflappable clinician. He has seen hundreds of trauma cases, strokes and cardiac arrests. He knows when someone needs to go to hospital and when they don't.
- Will is halfway through his specialist paramedic course. He is learning (quickly) that the past 10 years have been spent dodging invisible bullets, and every new condition he learns about scares him.

Activity

Where do you fit on the scale from Table 6.1: Levels of Expertise? Where would you plot yourself on the Dreyfus Scale? Can you relate this to any experiences you've had or decisions you've made in practice or on placement?

Think carefully about each feature and before reading on, make your own judgement on the cases of Stacey, Jameel and Will using Table 6.2. Then add your own experiences in the row at the bottom.

Table 6.2 Example Table for Assessing Examples on the Dreyfus Scale

Paramedic	Score from Table 6.1	Dreyfus Scale
Stacey		
Jameel		
Will		
You		

How did you get on? Is there actually a correct answer to this? Perhaps not – so just compare your feelings to the answers in the completed Table 6.3 and consider the justifications given for each paramedic and see if you agree.

Table 6.3 Assessment of the Scenarios Using the Dreyfus Scale

Paramedic	Score from Table 6.1	Dreyfus Scale	Justification
Stacey	1 – I don't know what I don't know	Novice	This paramedic is overconfident and thinks that there is no more to learn. She also lacks experience and consolidation in practice.
Jameel	1 – I don't know what I don't know	Ad-vanced beginner	This paramedic has misplaced his experience for knowledge and has probably been rather lucky so far, rather than skillful.
Will	2 - I know what I don't know	Novice	This paramedic has reset the clocks and gone back to school to become a specialist paramedic. In this context he is a novice again, but he has the insight to know what he doesn't know.
Your self-assessment			

This exercise is an oversimplification but highlights the fact that experience does not necessarily confer competency.

When it comes to experience, you will meet colleagues on your travels who make statements extolling their brilliance by dint of decades of experience – 'I have been doing this job for 30 years, mate', or similar assertions, usually peppered with embellished tales of 'derring-do'. Without wanting to denigrate 30 years of dedicated service to patients, it is still appropriate to ask what those 30 years meant in reality. Let's put it this way: if you walk to work using the same route every day for a year, can you say you have an extra year's worth of experience of making journeys on foot? Could you therefore infer from this experience that this made you a better walker or navigator? Of course not. You have simply walked the same walk dozens of times following on from the very first day when you learned the route. Similarly, make sure that you can account for your clinical experiences by satisfying yourself that you haven't repeated the same one over and over without learning from it. Experience requires consolidation and learning before you even consider applying it intuitively. Even then, relying on intuition is risky.

In the film *Groundhog Day*, the character Phil (played by Bill Murray) has been given a gift from which all clinicians would benefit once in their careers. He is able to completely mess up every experience on that given day, time and time and time again, each time trying something different to improve the outcome. For instance, he had no idea that Rita likes French poetry – how could he have known on day one? After several attempts, though, he learns a poem which captivates her, thereby moving her emotionally towards his ultimate goal. This play on how experience is gained and consolidated is a great example for clinicians – particularly when you contrast the intuitive approach Phil takes early on in the film with his later actions. As he gains experience, he learns what works and what doesn't.

Experience, therefore, is useful rather than essential. We should try to quantify what experience is when we consider relying on it. Remember the pitfalls that come with using intuition or experience in isolation. When standing on the precipice of a clinical decision that will affect a real-life patient, that is more complex than you realize. Imagine yourself as the BASE jumper. Are you going to jump today because it was OK on the previous one hundred emergency calls, or do you use your consolidated knowledge, skill, judgement and experience to think of other options?

Judgement and Sense-making

There is more than one way to reach a destination.

This final section provides a brief overview of judgement, and making sense of the decisions we make as paramedics within the complex, real world of healthcare. As with the Toronto Transit Commission (TTC), there are many ways to reach the same destination. Does this mean that there is always an optimal decision?

For instance, reaching a destination on the TTC, there may be a direct route, a quick route but with changes, or an easy-to-remember route. One notable example on the TTC is choosing a route to Bloor and Yonge from Kennedy; on the TTC map there are a couple of choices. However, with enough thought the most direct and quickest route may be to Uber (complex or heuristic). Of course, if there is heavy automobile traffic, Uber may not be suitable and the preference may then shift to a TTC route.

The shifting dynamics of the real world render it very difficult to make an optimal decision. In a paramedic context this can cause a divergence in thinking. Examples include:

1. A child who's fallen off a swing and bruised an arm. Is this case simple or complex to you?
2. A chronic productive cough and a history of smoking. Depending on your role, what next steps might you take?
3. An unexpected death found after >15 minutes with no resuscitation effort. Does this require complex thinking?
4. A NEWS2 score wavering between 4 and 5. Does this need a pre-alert?

However, using the cognitive continuum enables clinicians to use judgement as to which path to take (intuitive/simple, deliberate/complex). This does not necessarily improve concurrence between clinicians and the decisions they make, though it does demonstrate a sound cognitive process that other individuals may be able to make sense of.

The concept of sense-making is a leadership skill that enables individuals to construct a framework that helps explain, interpret and extrapolate a situation into a comprehensible idea that others can understand (Weick, 2005; Weick, 1995). An easy formula to remember this process is:

Information → Schema → Insight → Product

(Pirolli and Card, 2005)

This formula represents similar ideas that were discussed in the previous chapter, where information can be thought of as patient history, signs and symptoms; schema as the hypotheses or ideas that form; insight as the clinician's capability as well as their awareness to error and risk; and product as the decision. The difference between decision-making and sense-making is that the former results in an action, whereas the latter is a contemplation. Sense-making in essence, is a form of reflection that can help reinforce a decision, which in turn can help rationalize decisions, particularly when there is discordance between clinicians or patients regarding a proposed management plan.

Furthermore, sense-making is applicable to the unknown (Ancona, 2012). Sometimes a paramedic is faced with an uncertain situation, a patient with a rare disease, for instance, with no obvious care plan in place. As in the previous chapter, it is okay to not know, so long as you rule out the concerning conditions, reduce any error, safety-net and refer appropriately. Admitting you don't know is always preferable to ignoring the fact you have no idea and hoping for the best.

A poignant example is during the early days of the Covid-19 pandemic, in which the disease presented wide and various symptoms (respiratory, flu-like, gastric, even chilblains), which rendered it difficult to differentiate amongst similar diseases, and often resulted in sudden deterioration. With few tests, overflowing hospitals, and primary care flooded with a concerned population, risk stratification became difficult. For paramedics, the closest ally was the sats probe, in combination with the NEWS2 score and thorough safety-netting, before any further guidance and tests would become apparent to aid decisions. Referring a patient became difficult due to the system-wide demand. Nevertheless, this offered paramedics an opportunity to make sense of the situation and take the lead in demonstrating the capability of the profession in courageously managing uncertainty in out-of-hospital care, but also disseminating lessons learned in delivering effective clinical decisions (see, for example, Rees et al., 2021; Higginson et al., 2020; Tang et al., 2020).

Making sense of uncertainty isn't solely for research paramedics or those leading the profession: any paramedic ought to reflect on the daily decisions they make, especially uncertain ones or those where there is a lack of concurrence – the essence of the garden gate test!

Think back to the way you processed information in the clinical scenario in Chapter 5 (p. 121), which highlighted the relationship between decisions and sense-making. A list of questions was put forward in order to determine a diagnosis. Abdominal pain is a useful example to use, as it is a notoriously difficult to get the diagnosis correct. In fact, the literature suggests that clinicians should expect to be wrong with the diagnosis 50% of the time (Simon et al., 2005). The most important point is that the process of making an accurate decision must be used, and you cannot simply walk away based on intuition or heuristic alone. If the patient in the example had been assessed using only intuition or experience, she might have been left at home with a potentially life-threatening condition.

Charlin et al. (2000) suggest that decision making based on information processing is made utilizing cycles of hypotheses and deduction in an iterative way, building and testing hypotheses from many sources. The case study involving Elliott demonstrates the cyclical nature of decision making and the importance of using process. It is important to know where to get the information from and to recognize the sources you can use to generate hypotheses. This is the point where sense-making intersects with the decision; there is a clear trend that Elliott is pregnant and further investigation is required. How this is managed with Elliott and her mother since there is now a conflict is arguably just as crucial in terms of patient care. By reflecting upon your insight as a paramedic, it may well be that you make the decision for Elliott and her mother to make their own way to hospital so they can have some privacy, or closely follow behind. Perhaps Elliott may wish to come alone in the ambulance. Had you considered there might be a safeguarding issue, for example, who and how old is the expectant father? Without reflection we cannot evolve our ideas, decisions or ability to communicate them to others.

So, what sources of information can be used to generate your hypotheses or schema? The main groups can be broken down into different lines of enquiry, such as:

- What the patient tells you.
- What the patient chooses not to tell you.
- What family members and carers tell you.
- Signs (e.g., skin colour).
- Symptoms (e.g., nausea).
- Diagnostic tests (e.g., ECG, blood glucose, blood pressure).
- Vomit, stool, urine.

In any scenario, this process can be repeated until you reach a point where you either find the answer, or you decide that you are unable to find the answer – your capability point. The graph in Figure 6.4 shows how you start with many hypotheses and, as you move toward the solution, the number of hypotheses reduces. Eventually, a hypothesis will stand out above the rest, or you are unable to cross the red-line threshold and remain uncertain. Either way, as a paramedic you will need to make sense and manage appropriately, effectively communicating these concerns

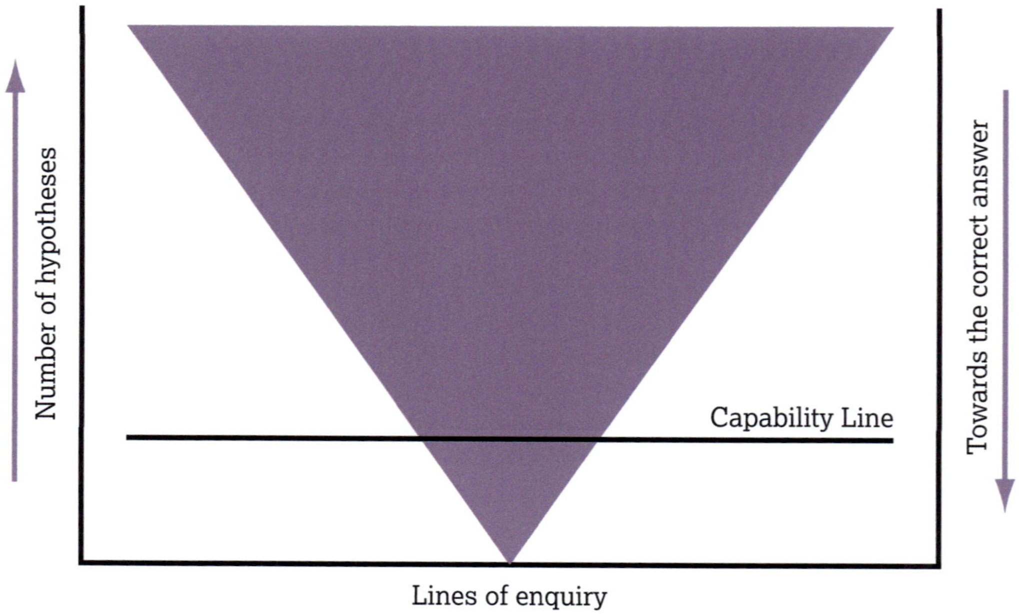

Figure 6.4 Hypotheses and solutions line.

with the patient. Typically, if the red line has not been crossed, you must refer to someone else.[2]

Conclusion

Passing the garden gate test requires you to have made a robust decision, which can be defended and explained. While the origins of the test arose from a scenario involving leaving a patient at home and not sending them to hospital, every decision has a garden gate regardless of the complexity of the scenario or acuity of the patient. The outcome of the test hinges on making sure you have addressed the 'why' as well as the 'what', and that any decisions stand up to your own reflective scrutiny.

There will always be times where you simply do not know what is wrong with the patient. Until such time as there are portable CT scanners and integrated point of care blood tests available, you will have to refer the patient for ongoing care to another clinical team. Bear in mind that the decision to refer patients is a decision in itself and must be approached with the same consideration.

Remember that you can use peers and senior colleagues to test your hypotheses, and the process of **shared decision making** is a very good way of enhancing patient safety. Do not mistake your autonomy as a pressure to work alone. Autonomy gives you freedom to think and freedom to act; choosing to seek advice and guidance does not make you a bad clinician and should not make you feel less autonomous. However, abdicating your decision making and sending all your patients to hospital would suggest a lack of autonomy and professional responsibility.

As you move from this chapter into the next, consider the decisions you make and the conclusions you draw. Think about the importance of each decision point – the fork in the road requiring you to take a particular route – and how difficult it is to track back once you have negotiated three or four major decisions in a row. The fact is that making good decisions is good for patients, and developing your professional practice means taking responsibility. Decision making skills require practice. You will move from novice to expert as long as you know what you know, and what you don't know.

This chapter set out to guide you on a path to becoming a better decision maker, showing you how to make sense of situations, particularly those involving conflict and uncertainty. The use of the cognitive continuum in knowing when to make a simple or complex decision was discussed, and the introduction of ways to understand what you know and what you don't know has been presented. The following chapter applies these aspects in greater detail, putting everything

[2] Although beyond the scope of this book, some diseases are very difficult to identify but nevertheless typically resolve with time or a standard treatment plan. Dermatological presentations (rashes) are an example of this, and dermatologist referrals generally occur after an initial treatment plan has failed. However, decisions such as this need to be made within the right competence and setting, with monitoring by the primary care team.

discussed in the previous chapters together and embedding them against the backdrop of the wider healthcare community.

Reflective Exercises

1. Pick a clinical condition you think you know well and try to develop a list of signs and symptoms that are associated with the condition. Then develop a list of hypotheses to test.
2. Reflect on the use of intuition in your personal and professional life. Consider when it matters and when it doesn't. Then consider times where you have acted intuitively – regardless of the outcome being correct or incorrect – and review your processing.
3. How do you perceive experience in practice? Reflecting on the novice to expert journey, how important is experience in comparison to effective structured decision making.
4. Think about a decision you were unsure of, perhaps one that was challenged by another clinician or patient. Given the reality of the situation, think about whether you were able to convey the rationale, and if you considered any suitable alternatives. With reflection, what might you have done differently?

Chapter 7

Refining and Improving the Application of Decision Making in Practice

Kieren Pugh and Andy Collen

Chapter Objectives

This chapter will cover:

- Consolidating your own experience
- Pre and post-test probability
- Feedback
- Considering professional risk and consequence
    - Mitigating risk: management vs avoidance
    - Documentation
    - Practising defensibly rather than defensively
- Considering sinister presentations
- Working together for your patient
    - Collaborative decision making
    - Reasonable decisions in practice
    - Differing opinions: managing professional conflict
- Balancing thoroughness and effectiveness with the needs of the wider population.

Introduction

Chapter 6: The Garden Gate Test discussed the ways in which we can avoid accumulating unresolved concerns resulting from our decisions. Making a good decision must also include mitigation against error, and there are strategies that can be used to help underpin each encounter to ensure your patient is safe, and your practice is not influenced by fear – rather, that it is bounded by an understanding of risks and is resolved in such a way that protects all concerned as far as possible.

This chapter explores a range of experiences and challenges you may face in practice, and the practical applications of decision-making techniques. Chapter 3 gave an overview of different decision-making theories and models, which will be drawn on here, as we explore how to recognize when your decision making is hampered and how best to mitigate risk.

Understanding errors and mistakes, and concepts such as collaborative decision making, will be touched upon to reflect the turning tide of culture in paramedic practice, which is essential for better patient care. Think about the section in the previous chapter about safety science, error management, and systems thinking, and how you operate in complex socio-technical healthcare settings.

To assist with navigating this chapter, read the case study below and consider the patient outlined therein. The learning points in this chapter will reference this patient in terms of how they present and the ways in which problems can be anticipated and overcome. The case study is followed by practical examples with reflective exercises at the end of the chapter, which will help you to reflect on your knowledge and assist with further developing your decision-making skills.

Case Example: Mo

You are working on an ambulance as a paramedic with a colleague and you are sent to an emergency call in the next town for a 45-year-old male with 'chest discomfort'. There is very little information available to you, but you establish the call has originated through the 811 service and been passed to 911 for an emergency response. You arrive at the address and are met with a globally well-looking male patient, complaining of chest discomfort. He is very keen to dismiss the fact that this is an emergency and apologizes for calling you out; he was, in fact, in the process of trying to stand the ambulance down, but the message had not filtered through. As you are already committed to scene, and have made contact with Mo, you offer him an assessment, which he accepts.

You gain a comprehensive history, establishing that the pain developed while Mo was lifting weights in the gym around two hours ago. It feels like an aching pain, 'like a sprained muscle' Mo tells you. It's localized to the right-hand side with no radiation, and it is reproduced by palpation. The patient is not primarily concerned about the level of pain, but rather was seeking to be pain free throughout the night and had sought advice about analgesia from the 811 service, who had passed the call to 911 as chest pain was described during triage.

The patient seems in good spirits and outwardly appears clinically well to you as you prepare to commence your physical examination. There is nothing visible upon inspection in terms of contusion or trauma on the skin. His medical history elicits generally good health with no ongoing illnesses, and he takes no medications. Socially, he lives an active lifestyle, he used to smoke 'like a train' in his early twenties but has since given up. He drinks occasionally but is not dependent on alcohol. His family history is not particularly concerning, with no unexplained cardiac events, heart disease or diabetes. He states, however, that his grandfather had 'high cholesterol'. His observations are reproduced in Table 7.1.

Table 7.1 Mo's Observations

Heart rate	90 per minute, regular (taken from pulse oximeter)
Respiratory rate	14 breaths per minute
Blood pressure	135/68 (taken on the patient's left arm with automated sphygmomanometer)
Temperature	37.0°C (tympanic thermometer)

You are comfortable after a discussion with your colleague that the patient does not require a 12-lead ECG after a diagnosis of 'obvious MSK chest pain' being made. Your differentials include costochondritis, pathological rib fracture and, at the more sinister end of the spectrum, stable pulmonary embolism, and acute coronary syndrome. Although you feel these are unlikely, you document them accordingly in the list of differential diagnoses.

With this evidence, you are confident in your diagnosis. You give the patient an informed choice of options and he opts to follow up with his NP for analgesia rather than being taken to ED. Mo is very grateful for your help and you leave the property and book clear with the ambulance communication centre.

Consolidating Your Own Experience

When considering the journey from novice to expert (Benner, 1984) and how clinicians in their early years may be influenced in their approach to problems based on factors such as their undergraduate education and the influence of peers/colleagues, the roles of practice education, supervision and mentorship become vital.

Being aware of the differences between deduction and experience-based pattern recognition is a key theme in this book and that awareness is an essential tool. Placing trust on intuition based on 'what you know you know', as we have seen, is quick and can be beneficial to the patient – especially if you have a large case load or you are working in a high-pressure situation. It is worth challenging yourself when you find you have made a decision through intuition rather than deduction in these busy situations. Ask yourself to 'prove' (to yourself!) that the diagnosis you have made is right, and reflect upon the process that you took to reach your decision. Analysing your thought process and decision can help to mitigate any cognitive biases that particularly impact on diagnostic process – **availability and confirmation bias**, specifically.

As we discussed in Chapter 6, more experienced clinicians may be able to rapidly gain new information, test, retest, validate and reject information. However, even though more experience may result in increased confidence for coming up with hypotheses and evaluating their specificity, this must also be underpinned by consideration for the patient, specifically their safety and experience, taking into account the risks of over-testing and delaying their care. We will discuss in more detail how testing plays a part in improving your decision making as a clinician.

Pre- and Post-test Probability

Performing tests may be such a routine part of your practice, that you may not have taken the time to reflect on the importance of selecting, performing and interpreting tests on the decision-making process. Testing has an important impact on your decision making, whether you carry out the test or not.

Tests in this sense can mean anything from a measurement of blood pressure to invasive procedures, such as blood capillary glucose monitoring. In hospital and primary care, they can range from serum blood tests to computed tomography (CT) scanning. All tests will have benefits and risks, and these must be weighed up and be communicated to the patient so that they understand why the tests are being proposed. Testing should always be in the patient's best interests and undertaken only to direct care, rather than to satisfy curiosity. Prior to carrying out the test, as with any healthcare intervention, you must ensure that the patient has the capacity to understand what is being proposed, and where capacity is lacking, you must work with carers or family members to advocate for the patient in context to the reason for testing and the potential distress the testing may cause.

Below are some questions you might ask yourself before undertaking a test:

- Do you understand why you want to do the test?
- What result are you expecting the test to show?
- What are you going to do if the test is positive?
- What are you going to do if the test is negative?
- Will the test result influence your treatment course?
- Can the test wait?

By way of example, in pre-hospital care, depending on the employer, there can be a tendency to complete a capillary blood glucose and temperature on every patient, regardless of whether it is relevant to the clinical decision or would influence any change of trajectory for the patient. Outside of planned screening programmes, testing blood glucose, temperature or blood pressure based on compliance rather than to promote patient safety or outcomes, could be seen as over-testing. While it could also provide an opportunity for a serendipitous finding, consideration should be given to the ethical and resource implications of this, and the role of primary care in managing disease at a population level. Therefore, the types of tests we carry out can also tie into aspects of cultural change; often when something has been done a certain way for so long, it becomes difficult to reverse that practice. People may say, 'We've always done it this way'.

Over-testing

Consider an example of a patient with an unusual presentation, so you decide to perform every test you can think of – blood tests, a CT scan, MRI scan – to find the answer. Were all of these tests really necessary?

The simple answer is 'no'. You will likely get the same answer as an expert practitioner, but you just took a longer way to get there. In the meantime, you would have also exposed the patient to potentially unnecessary radiation, pain and infection risks by **over-testing**. Reflecting on the importance of giving patients the opportunity to make an informed choice, selecting relevant tests becomes part of your broader clinical and professional acumen, weaving together patient factors and your ongoing plan of care.

Unnecessary investigations can be a burden: this includes the financial burden to the organization as a whole, the emotional burden on the patient awaiting a result they didn't need, and unwarranted workload for laboratories or other clinicians (O'Sullivan et al., 2018). Above everything else is knowing what to do with any result you receive, whether expected or not. Not only do we need to consider why we might be undertaking a test, but also consider our information processing and subsequent rationale. Serendipitous diagnoses are a wonderful event when they occur, but by their very nature are uncovered by chance rather than by intent. This is where an entirely unrelated disease process is found during an encounter for another presentation. For example, while taking a history on a patient with a turned ankle in an Urgent Treatment Centre, you notice a sinister lesion on the patient's head, which then leads to a two-week wait referral for a suspected carcinoma. The lesion is removed before it can spread, and the patient's life is saved. Their ankle fracture also heals well.

The point to reflect on when we draw together practical and ethical considerations is that over-testing and screening is not necessarily the correct course of action, although a level of vigilance and willingness to make serendipitous diagnoses is a positive trait. Consider the impact on availability of you as a healthcare resource if you screened all patients who present with a turned ankle for skin cancer. The numbers needing treatment would be huge, and the impact on patients waiting would be significant, regardless of the practice setting you are in.

Think back to Mo's case at the beginning of the chapter; the decision was made to omit performing a 12-lead ECG on this patient. We are *expecting* the result to be normal (due perhaps to confirmation bias). Would the same clinical course be taken if the result is negative, and would it influence the treatment course? Are we confident with our diagnosis, as the patient is not displaying a classical cardiac picture?

Had a 12-lead ECG have been completed – a 'positive result' – it would have shown **anterior ST segment elevation**. This patient was suffering from a dissecting aorta. Relevant to aortic dissection is the report by the HSIB in 2020 (HSIB, 2020) regarding delays that a patient with a dissecting aneurysm experienced, leading to harm. The patient in the HSIB report was taken to a non-specialist hospital and spent some hours awaiting the diagnosis, and the report highlighted a general lack of awareness that was found in this case with aortic dissection and its non-standard features. Mo may have been having a heart attack and therefore the ECG findings are not definitive in this respect. Again, consideration has to be given to accessing investigations that can provide a diagnosis and transferring the patient there versus what you need to know in your context (i.e., primary care clinical consulting room or ambulance).

This highlights that, while being confident with your diagnosis is essential, so is being aware of the 'unknown unknowns'. It is an extreme but realistic example, and not every patient with musculoskeletal chest pain would receive a 12-lead ECG either in pre-hospital practice, hospital practice, or in primary care – but the potential exists for sinister pathology as described earlier.

When reflecting on the four pillars of biomedical ethics discussed in Chapter 2 (autonomy, beneficence, non-maleficence, justice), what problems do over-testing present? Patient expectations are pivotal, and the medico-legal implications of a missed diagnosis can cause anxiety and moral injury for healthcare professionals. Caregivers do not seek to cause harm and may themselves become 'second victims' (Dekker, 2013) following patient harm events they are involved in (which include diagnostic, treatment and management errors). It is worth reflecting that, as our profession grows and sees more patients in different settings with different pressures and risk profiles, our own psychological wellbeing, as well as promoting patient safety and outcomes, becomes a bigger issue. The backdrop to this is that patients are becoming more complex (i.e., due to multi-morbidity, polypharmacy), which makes all aspects of care more challenging. This may perhaps lead to a greater risk of over-testing in light of a perceived greater risk of misdiagnosis. Strategies can be developed to assist, such as CPD, governance activities, clinical supervision, clinical audit, service development, patient satisfaction surveying and professional feedback, among others, and these can help to reduce the feeling of isolation in practice. Fundamentally, though, two heads are better than one – always seek support.

Feedback

It is generally seen as a positive if a clinician 'hasn't heard anything back' about their healthcare encounters, and this may be considered a proxy for not being wrong; this can therefore often be the sole determinant of disposition success. However, we know that feedback loops in clinical practice as a whole, let alone paramedic practice, are poor (Pollard and Black, 2015). The literature also looks differently at learning through processes such as appreciative inquiry, which explores when things have gone well and is similar to the principle of Safety 2 (Hollnagel et al., 2015), which is used in safety-critical industries (see Chapter 4). Some innovative schemes have also been set up around the UK to feedback to paramedics who work in an ambulance service setting, to update them on a diagnosis and treatment pathway for their patients. The way this works is by 'closing the loop' of feedback to a clinician after their journey with a patient has finished through a process of structured clinical feedback provided to the clinician/crew. These schemes differ in terms of process, but all share the core function of allowing paramedics and ambulance crews to find out what happened to their patient.

These systems also raise the need to clarify what should be fed back in terms of impact on the clinician, relating to the potential for psychological harm versus the benefits for learning. For example, what would be the impact on the paramedic knowing that you had made an incorrect diagnosis about a patient who was taken to the correct hospital in terms of raising the importance of diagnostic certainty versus fundamentally safe care. Sadly, the laws that protect patient information also stifle patient level feedback for paramedics and we commonly lack the justification to review patient outcomes as we usually have no ongoing direct care. The ability to gain consent from the patient to share information about their outcome is often unrealistic, particularly in the emergency setting, where consent to share information would be sought at a time where the patient may be under duress and therefore the consent may not be valid.

Feedback can be easier for colleagues working in primary care who may receive discharge information on their registered patients, although time constraints and simply remembering which patients you saw would also be challenging. All healthcare settings face challenges in organizing governance and supervision for staff, as well as having the resources to set up patient surveys, although many overcome these and perform better for doing so.

The benefits of feedback can be far reaching; for example, personal reflection and peer review discussion are just some of the advantages. These are not only beneficial to our own progression and mental wellbeing, but also have positive impacts on patient safety and outcomes. We operate in systems where compliance is often valued over skill, feedback, audit, governance, peer review and other kinds of continuous learning. Assurance and compliance may be perceived as effective oversight by system leaders charged with important and necessary regulatory focus, but should be balanced with professional activities that holistically support good care, and which in turn improves regulatory compliance. Arguably, feedback is a condition of learning. When we think about concepts such as heuristics, those learned skills and subroutines are based on continuous feedback. Your decision-making skills will benefit from embracing all forms of feedback and, as healthcare professionals, we should inform and control these activities as part of our growth and learning.

Considering Professional Risk and Consequence

Mitigating Risk: Management *vs* Avoidance

Healthcare is a risky business. Patients deserve the very best care, and this must be delivered in a safe way. It is simply unrealistic, however, to manage every condition by referring to a hospital consultant or putting the patient through a barrage of tests. Most health conditions that occur spontaneously (illness) or are acquired (injury) are self-limiting, or need only minor interventions to correct them; yet some are cryptic, occult, atypical or overlaid upon a complex health history. For some patients, illness and injury are compounded by extremes of age, social and economic circumstance, or capacity to care for oneself. Against this backdrop, we are expected to reduce the impact on our wider health and social care systems.

Safe care is not about taking risks, it is about understanding risks and seeking to mitigate as far as is reasonable. Sadly, things do not always run to plan and patients can deteriorate unexpectedly or suffer a new, separate health emergency. When this happens – particularly when it leads to an investigation – it can have a deleterious effect on the confidence of the clinician who last cared for the patient with the unfavourable outcome, as well as that of the patient.

Human beings are, as we know, easily influenced by biases and fallacies. In his book, *Risk: The Science and Politics of Fear* (2009), Dan Gardner explores the impact the perception of risk had on Americans after the September 11 terrorist attacks in 2001. The American (and worldwide) public developed a greater fear of terrorism and perceived there to be a much greater risk of dying in a similar attack. As a result, many Americans stopped flying, choosing instead to drive interstate. As a result, it is estimated that an additional 1,600 people died in vehicle accidents in the years after 9/11. The risk of dying in an automobile accident versus dying in a terrorist attack was significantly higher, but due to the proximity and availability of the perceived threat, behaviours were altered with tragic consequences.

Documentation

One of the most important aspects of risk mitigation is documentation. Making a contemporaneous record of each healthcare encounter is essential in ensuring what happened was recorded and can be revisited in the future as necessary (see Figure 7.1). It is a commonly used quotation that always bears repeating:

> *If it isn't written down, it didn't happen.*

Keep accurate records of your work

You must keep full, clear and accurate records for everyone you care for, treat or provide other service to. You must complete all records promptly and as soon as possible after providing care, treatment or other services.

Full, clear and accurate record keeping is vital to the delivery of safe and effective healthcare

Once you are registered with us, you have a professional responsibility to keep full, clear and accurate records for everyone you care for, treat or provide other services to. This is to:

- safeguard continuity of care by providing information to colleagues involved in care and treatment;
- ensure service users receive appropriate treatment that is in their best interests;
- meet legal requirements or respond to Freedom of Information or Subject Access Requests; and
- evidence your decision-making processes if later queried or investigated.

What records you need to keep, in what format and for how long, varies depending on the setting you are working in and the subject matter of those records.

Figure 7.1 Keeping records of your work.
Source: HCPC, 2021

Structured documentation will help you to defend your practice, should this ever be necessary. More importantly it ensures that you prevent harm coming to your patient. Therefore, perhaps instead of perceiving the aspects of practice you employ to 'cover yourself', change your perspective and view these activities as those which make your care as safe as possible for your patient. For paramedics, and in fact all healthcare professionals, discharging a patient from care is probably the activity that carries the greatest perception of risk by clinicians, and is the reason the 'garden gate test' was developed. It is a fact that some patients will worsen, and/or the diagnosis/treatment given was incorrect. To err is human, and while we have argued in this book that diagnosis is merely a categorization task, sometimes even the best clinicians make errors. Therefore, it is not the act of discharging a patient in good faith and with adequate safety netting that represents the most risk – it is failing to consider the worst-case scenario and mitigating against it.

There are many models for structuring documentation, and some organizations provide pre-formatted and/or pre-printed patient advice leaflets to support the advice given verbally to patients. The list provided below is a suggested format for structuring written clinical records. These can be completed concisely, and need not take very long, but must cover the key areas discussed with the patient. Remember, these should reflect a conversation with the patient, and not exist solely as documentation in isolation.

Worsening Care Advice (WCA)

This is a list of 'what ifs' – the signs and symptoms that may be encountered by the patient (or witnessed by friends of family) and that may then require a follow-up action, which should also be documented and communicated to the patient/family/carer. For example, a patient who has back pain should expect the pain to remain quite constant and ease gradually over the coming days. The WCA discussed with the patient would involve a change in the pattern of pain, and include the red flags for cauda equina.

Safety Netting

Safety Netting was introduced into primary care some years ago, and there is a lack of consensus on what it must include. Therefore, the suggestion to use it in combination with WCA and LICO (see below) is an interpretation of its application in practice, which focuses on the specific 'what to do' advice in response to the WCA. For example, the patient with back pain should be advised that if they still have pain in several weeks (as is common with non-traumatic back pain), they should approach their GP. However, if they experience the signs and symptoms of cauda equina, they should immediately seek urgent follow up. Safety netting may be specific and include calling 811 or 911.

Left in Care of (LICO)

This aspect of documentation records who will be caring for the patient in the immediate period after their discharge (or while waiting for referral). For some patients this won't be necessary, but for others it won't be an option. Where a friend, family member, carer or neighbour is prepared to provide some after-care, it is important to document this, and include the patient's consent for this to happen. For example, you may document: 'Left in care of neighbour, who will sit with the patient until their daughter arrives. The patient has consented to this, and the WCA has been discussed with them'.

Documentation is a contemporaneous record of the encounter between you and your patient, and while it may never again see the light of day after being written, it remains a part of the patient's health record and is retained for at least 7–10 years for adults, and many more years for children. Remember to make your written records well structured, and use them to promote patient safety as a record of what you have advised your patient. This applies in all practice settings and, while it is most important when ending an episode of care (as opposed to taking a patient to the emergency department), consistent structured clinical documentation is a practised skill, which healthcare professionals must consider a cornerstone of practice that keeps patients safe and clinicians confident.

Practising Defensibly, Rather Than Defensively

The prospect of managing risk can be somewhat daunting and it is important that clinicians develop clear strategies to ensure that the responsibility of professional practice doesn't overwhelm or create unnecessary pressure, which may in turn lead to worse care for the patient.

As discussed earlier in the book, it is important to differentiate between **defensive practice** and practising **defensibly.** It is the sad reality that healthcare professionals fear consequence disproportionally and may alter their practice in response to the perceived need to avoid events that could lead to be being struck off.

There is a significant difference between defensible practice and defensive practice, and the methods you choose to use to promote safe practice for your patient and yourself should be proportional.

Defensive

- Used or intended to defend or protect.
- Very anxious to challenge or avoid criticism.

Defensible

- Justifiable by argument.
- Able to be protected.

Many of the synonyms associated with the word defensible are common to decision making, such as: justifiable, arguable, tenable, defendable, maintainable, sustainable, supportable, plausible, well founded, sound, sensible, reasonable, rational, logical.

Practising defensively can be influenced by a local investigation outcome or previous experiences and can negatively impact future patient encounters. A good example of this would be an occasion when you are called to a nursing home where a resident is said to have had a fall. They have a history of osteoporosis, and their head came into contact with the wall on falling. The patient has been assisted up off the floor by staff and you attend the patient some hours after the injury. You transport the patient to the local emergency department where it later transpires that they suffered a high cervical spine fracture from the fall. You did not minimize movement and consider the c-spine in the patient on this occasion, and, despite no harm coming to that patient, in the coming weeks you find yourself now being excessively sensitive with many of the uninjured fallers that you go to in the fear of missing an injury on another patient

– potentially risking overtreating or making care less comfortable. Perpetuating a range of biases can create unnecessary stress and anxiety, and can impact on other patients' care. The likelihood of a particular disease or injury is based on an individual patient, their health history and their presentation. We may neglect the base-rate following an adverse event, and so we need to consider the true likelihood of every patient we see having a certain injury in the absence of supporting clinical signs and symptoms.

Practising in this way is not helpful for yourself as the clinician (i.e., increased stress and worry about similar patient presentations and concern about colleagues questioning your abilities) and neither is it beneficial for patients who are unnecessarily immobilized and may undergo investigations that are not needed – (refer to over-testing on pp. 157–158).

The phrase 'covering your back' is sometimes used within healthcare; however, if you practise defensibly, and do the right thing, there is no need to consider 'your back' or, in the case of the registrant, your registration. Practising defensibly is having the ability to rationalize your decision making and having a rationale that is evidence based and documented. This means making a decision that is made with all the information available to you, weighing up the patient's wishes, interests, ideas and concerns, and following the medical model for patient history.

Considering Sinister Presentations

As discussed in Chapter 6 (p. 142–147), experience (chronological or episodic) is not absolutely essential in the formation of hypotheses, but experience in practice does serve to speed up the process of hypothesis generation. Remembering that creating a hypothesis is not in itself a decision; hypothesis generation is arguably a good place to allow your intuition to be exploited.

Practice is influenced by a number of different factors, such as the 'work as done', environment, organizational policy and culture. A mnemonic HALT is useful to note when you might be feeling the strains of intrinsic and extrinsic factors, standing for being **H**ungry, **A**ngry, **L**ate/**L**onely or **T**ired (Ragau et al., 2018). Safety-critical industries have learned that human performance degrades over time on duty, and this can be caused not just by tiredness or other human-related factors. Poor work design and ergonomics/environment can have a big impact on performance. If one (or all) of these are affecting you on a given day, performance and decisions may well be affected as a result. When we apply this specifically to a task such as making a diagnosis, the end result can be swayed or incorrect. For example, developing a list of differential diagnoses at the end of your shift may be harder than the ones you might make earlier in the shift with the same patient presentation. Cognitive bias (availability or confirmation) has already been spoken about. Something that became a bias during the Covid-19 pandemic was 'breathing problems' being attributed to Coronavirus without considering other diagnoses, and this was compounded by other changes in practice that created barriers between clinicians and patients, such as PPE and remote consultations.

A consistent theme throughout this book is the importance of approaching decisions based on structured enquiry, using methods to test, retest, reject or accept each theory, considering dynamically how other complex factors drive the process that leads to the correct outcome. Consider, then, how dismissing a patient with challenging behaviour on the basis of *what* they are outwardly displaying (as opposed to finding out *why* they present like this and missing a sinister problem) could lead to a poor outcome and experience for the patient. Again, considering that diagnosis is a categorization task, the risk of miscategorizing a patient's needs becomes ethically questionable if safeguards are not put in place, such as worsening care advice and safety netting. Therefore, the hypothesis becomes ever more important as a step on the way to the decision you make, and the subsequent onward decisions for treatment, referral and management. As with all things that involve human beings, we can be wrong – even if we use the correct approach, process and methods.

To expand on this further, beyond an acute behaviour change, most diagnoses will have a broad set of differentials behind them. Some will be very common, others not so. Think about a time where anchoring, availability or other bias played a part in the assessment of a patient. Below is a list of 'dangerous diagnoses' linked to common symptoms in practice. Be sure you have considered all possible alternatives before making these diagnoses, as they frequently can be attributed to other sinister causes (Hopcroft and Forte, 2020; Johnson and Hill-Smith, 2006):

- Anxiety (PE, MI)
- Covid-19 (LVF, sepsis, PE, ACS)
- Infection of the urinary tract (delirium, metabolic disturbance)
- Muscular skeletal chest pain (vascular emergency, PE, MI)
- Intoxication (head injury, stroke, metabolic disturbance, illicit substances)
- Gastroenteritis (acute abdominal pathology).

It is worth noting these diagnoses and being sure you have considered all others before settling on your decision outwardly. These diagnoses can present as fairly straightforward and innocuous, but we must recognize our limitations in practice, in whichever setting we may work, and the problems associated with limited clinical testing and access to senior support.

Working Together for Your Patient

Collaborative Decision Making

Due to the very nature of the work that paramedics do, the job can be very isolated, and it can be lonely making decisions by yourself at all hours of the day and night. Indeed, 'lone wolf' decision making isn't healthy for you or the patient. Sharing this cognitive load with a remote clinician can help remove some of the burden of making difficult decisions. Further to this, the importance of sharing the decision with a patient who is the expert on their own condition should not be underestimated to ensure we make every contact count.

Sharing the decisions we make for, and with, our patients, either between the clinician and patient (most commonly referred to as 'shared decision making' (NHS England, 2019b), or by augmenting decisions by discussing with a colleague ('collaborative or joint decision making', sometimes called 'shared *professional* decision making' (NHS England, n.d.a), is very important because it helps to mitigate potential risk and promotes patient activation and empowerment. As already discussed, making a good decision must also include mitigation against error, and there are strategies that can be used to help underpin each encounter to ensure your patient is safe and your practice is not influenced by fear – rather that it is bounded by an understanding of risks, and is resolved in such a way that protects all concerned as far as possible. Part of this process is shared or collaborative decision making – making sure patients understand what you have found, what you are proposing to do and what might happen next. Seeking understanding from your patient (where their capacity allows) greatly enhances the approach to risk. While decisions made with a patient must be done in light of good information (and that responsibility ultimately sits with the clinician), the patient who understands and consents to the course of action is the first line of defence regarding anticipated issues and ensuring they seek help.

For example, when we discharge a patient, this is the disposition with the most risk. That is because often there is no follow up to their care, and there may not be any onward referral to another healthcare professional who will then take responsibility for that patient's care. Therefore, the patient must be part of the discussion to ensure that they understand the factors that determine their own health following your encounter with them.

In paramedic practice, it is a privilege to meet a lot of patients who often have little contact with other services, and it may well be that we are the first healthcare professionals to be invited into their home for some time. This makes their discharge decision and safety netting even more important to consider and implement to ensure that encounter helps keep the patient connected with services and to optimize their physical and mental health (NHS England & Public Health England, 2016).

It would be unwise to omit reference to the patients for whom capacity is diminished, and the occasions where decisions are made in the best interest of a patient. The hypothetico-deductive model may be affected by the patient's capacity to understand questions. On occasion this may lead to a more clinically diagnostic approach, rather than through considering the health history primarily. For example, the unconscious patient cannot tell you why they are unconscious, and may not have any clues about their person to guide the decision. Therefore, you will look to the common causes as hypotheses (e.g., hypoglycaemia, intoxication) and exclude or confirm accordingly. Where the cause is hypoglycaemia, a blood glucose test can be obtained (in the patient's best interest) to confirm the cause, and this then allows treatment to be focused. This is a very simple example of capacity being diminished acutely and temporarily, and it is important that clinicians understand the principles associated with decision making involving patients who may lack capacity.

Historically, clinicians may have felt under pressure to work alone and not seek help with their decision making. It is hoped that perceptions are changing and there is now more help than there ever was to assist with getting the decision right first time. Clinical support paramedics (in Nova Scotia) or base hospital physicians (in Ontario) are examples of resources available to support decision making. Many reasons are cited for professionals not wanting to engage in discussions with other colleagues or the patients themselves for the right outcome, including workload pressure and lack of time. Often, the opinion also seems to come from not wanting to appear 'silly' or confessing that you don't know the answer to something. This is the joy of being a paramedic; there is a vast array of conditions, presentations and pathologies that you won't know about. When you come across a problem to which you don't know the answer, the safest thing for your patient, you as the healthcare professional and your organization is to find someone who does. Calling on a specialist in the area you are seeking help for ensures the best outcome for all involved.

Thinking back to discharge, if you take a foundation-year doctor who has undergone five years of undergraduate medical training, they will very likely be discussing discharge and referrals with their registrar or consultant. Why should it be any different for paramedics? A great benefit for those paramedics working in the community is that you will have a wealth of expertise around you to help decide outcomes and share decisions.

The ambulance service paramedic is, in contrast, somewhat more isolated. They will have access to clinicians on the telephone, often specialists in urgent care, to assist with referral and discharge decisions. The benefit of a remote opinion is far reaching: they will be able to consider the patient presentation from an angle that you may not have considered, offer alternative pathway advice and sometimes teach you about a rare condition. It is worth bearing in mind the complex medical presentations we are expected to assess, treat and diagnose with the little diagnostic equipment at our disposal, and sometimes a relative lack of knowledge of the condition you are treating links back to the 'unknown unknowns' (see Maslow).

Specific to ambulance service practice, the decision to convey a patient to hospital has been seen as the 'safe' option and provides an assumed failsafe if you are unsure. Arguably practice is on the verge of change, as clinicians are having more detailed discussions about their conveyance decisions with a range of other clinicians. Paramedics are acutely aware of the risks of avoidable prolonged admission (delirium, loss of muscle mass, decreases in functional ability), and these should be weighed up against the risks of receiving care in the community. Obviously, it goes without saying that there is a group of patients and diagnoses for which hospital admission is unequivocal. Further, delaying an inevitable hospital admission until the next day or the next crew is also counterproductive. The facts to consider and the questions to ask yourself are:

- Is there anybody else that can care for this patient here at home?
- Am I making the decision (to convey or not to convey) for myself or for the patient?
- Is it reasonable to explore alternative pathways/treatment with a specialist?

Reasonable Decisions in Practice

> Reasonableness: Based on or using good judgement and therefore fair and practical.
>
> (Cambridge Dictionary, 2021)

In wider medicine, and indeed in paramedic practice, we talk about how 'reasonable' a decision is. A reasonable decision is one based on good judgement.

An example of a reasonable clinical decision would be the discussion of the appropriateness of discharging a patient in a nursing home who has rolled out of bed with a head injury. The patient takes anticoagulants and is approaching the end of life; a risk–benefit discussion and a conversation about the likely outcomes and interventions with due consideration to the clinical practice guidelines and evidence would be a good example of reasonableness. All of these factors combined with the patient's wishes, advance care planning documentation and family opinions help us to arrive at the best outcome.

Broadly speaking, an 'unreasonable' decision would be a discharge of a patient in their 40s on anticoagulants with a head injury after falling from a ladder and with no advance decisions made or near the latter stages of any end-stage disease trajectory. In practice, there are multiple factors at play here, which have been discussed throughout this book.

The 'grey' and difficult areas of practice are where paramedics thrive the most, adapting and overcoming problems, finding pragmatic solutions to problems that present as an emergency. This is why it can sometimes be difficult for someone remote from the situation to see the 'reasonableness' of a decision, and where the 'wisdom of the crowd' can be useful – seeking the opinion of other professionals to see what their opinion is. This also links back to the importance of collaborative decision making with specialists and other healthcare professionals.

The 'Bolam test' came about in the 1950s after a medical negligence hearing (Eaton, 2024). The principle of the Bolam test is that a healthcare professional is not deemed 'negligent' if they abide by the standard of a responsible body of medical opinion. It can be used by healthcare professionals as a benchmark for what is acceptable among other colleagues to judge if care in a specific case was acceptable or not. This is despite there being differing bodies of evidence.

In practice, if the decision or task undertaken was judged by a group of the same professionals to be acceptable, then the practitioner is not negligent (Hurwitz, 2004).

Approaching Professional Conflict and Encouraging Challenge

Inevitably there will be times where there are differing thoughts about the plan that best meets the patient's needs. This is common throughout our practice, and indeed medicine as a whole, and is overwhelmingly good practice to discuss any differentiation. Once it is identified that professionals have different opinions about what to do for a patient – making sure patient safety is not compromised is the first priority. Thinking back to Chapter 4 and the Tenerife air disaster, graded assertiveness can help with this and there are a few strategies and approaches that can help you with this. It may be that the patient is so unwell that immediate action needs to be taken and that there is little time to discuss options; a debrief can happen later in these cases. In most other scenarios exploring the ideas and concerns of the other people on scene, including the patient and family, is useful. Being honest about your worries – for example, deterioration, lack of safety netting or co-morbidities – prompting you to transport to hospital will hopefully reassure your colleague that secondary care is appropriate for this patient. Similarly, listening to everyone's views in turn can change an initial plan that you had for the patient and improve the quality of the encounter.

The PACE model is an example of graded assertiveness. PACE stands for:

- Probe – asking questions, such as 'what procedure are we doing today?'
- Alert – using phrases, such as 'just checking that you have seen that the patient is contraindicated for that drug'.
- Challenge – making statements, such as 'I think this is the wrong thing to do and I am concerned – can we pause to recheck?'
- Escalate – using directive phrases, such as 'I am going to include the consultant, as you have not considered my concerns.'

Apply this to the case of Elaine Bromiley, which was mentioned in Chapter 3. After watching the film, consider which elements of PACE were used and which were not used. How would you have used PACE in this case?

- Web Link: *'Just a Routine Operation'* https://www.youtube.com/watch?v=JzlvgtPlof4

Balancing Thoroughness and Effectiveness with the Needs of the Wider Population

Healthcare is, as we have discussed throughout this book, a complex, safety-critical industry, which has to manage lots of risks, moving parts and uncertainty in an ever more financially challenged and publicly scrutinized manner. In almost all areas of healthcare, capacity tries to keep up with demand, and clinicians are required to manage their work rate and be aware of themselves as a precious resource. This is vital for the patient as well as their own wellbeing.

It would be prudent to explore some practice-based examples of this practical conundrum that paramedics must increasingly face. Many other healthcare professionals routinely use a 'make own way to ED' approach when dealing with their caseload. However, historically in the ambulance service this was seen as a controversial thing to do, although practice and policy are evolving in this aspect of care. What we mean in this context is that when a clinician has assessed a patient as needing further care and investigation, but without the need for ongoing monitoring and/or intervention, they may ask the patient to make their own way to hospital. This serves two purposes that are mutually exclusive; the decision is correct for that patient's ongoing care and the ambulance is available to attend another patient. This supports the ethical principle that we have a responsibility to ensure that our skills and resources are available to those who need them. This will involve dynamic decision making, much like instances where multiple patients are present, and a decision needs to be made around who requires your help first.

At first glance it might be observed that the ambulance service has always been seen as the service that deals with acute emergencies and so it would never be reasonable to explore alternative dispositions other than for the ambulance to convey the patient. However, we know that paramedic practice and indeed paramedic workload has changed dramatically in recent years. No longer is the ambulance service reserved for 'just' emergencies; we are expected to, and do, deal with undifferentiated urgent and primary care issues, chronic health problems and the exacerbations of these. To this end, as demand begins to rise for our services, other patients begin to wait longer for an ambulance response. Demand is growing exponentially every year and in the absence of managing this demand at the point of call connect, we need to ensure we can be available for patients when they need us. A thought to consider helping with this point is to think about your **task-cycle time.**

> **Task-cycle time** is the time taken to complete one patient encounter and be subsequently available for the next.

For example, you are called to see a 10-year-old child with a fever and right-sided abdominal pain. On examination there is abdominal tenderness and a fever with associated vomiting. The patient is otherwise clinically well, with normal observations, and no sign of systemic compromise. You know that this patient needs ED investigation to rule out possible appendicitis. You spend 25 minutes on scene assessing and writing paperwork, you transport them on the 30-minute journey to hospital, spend 15 minutes handing over and cleaning the back of the ambulance, before being available for the next call. An alternative to this disposition would have been asking if the parents were happy to transport the patient to the ED – obviously, this could only be done if organizational policy and authority allows, and if it was assessed as safe and appropriate for that patient and their family. This way, you are now clear to attend the next emergency call in half the time you would have been ordinarily, in a rural area with sparse ambulance cover. It also means you are available to serve the wider waiting community, one of which could be a cardiac arrest that you are currently in close proximity to. It is difficult to manage public perception, as paramedics who arrive on ambulances have the transporting capability. However, it is an important part of our role as healthcare professionals to educate, and to debunk myths that arriving at hospital by ambulance will not necessarily ensure you are 'seen quicker'.

The decision to discuss with patients and/or their family transporting themselves to hospital is perfectly reasonable, and the barriers around this would benefit from being broken down and questioned. The threshold for encouraging a 'make own way' approach should always be in the patient's best interests and not your own. For example, do you envisage any deterioration en-route? Do you anticipate any intervention by you en-route? If the answers to both these questions are 'no', then it is usually acceptable for a relative to transport the patient. Colleagues in primary care and other settings are well-versed in doing this. The benefit of working in an ED or in a GP setting is the 'waiting room effect' where we can see how many patients are waiting for our services. This could have an impact on our decision making, as the busier we see the waiting room, the more inclined we may be to work quicker. In an ambulance service setting, you might hear 'broadcasts' for high-acuity calls, but do you ever hear one for the uninjured older person who falls and has been on the floor for some time?

Accurate and contemporaneous documentation is essential to managing the risk for patients' onward care and as a 'look-back' should this be needed. A plan and rationale for your decision making at the time is invaluable for anyone retrospectively looking at treatment or outcome. For example, the advice that you give them on what to do if their condition should get worse. Also useful is paraphrasing the conversations you had with other healthcare professionals to decide on the most appropriate course of action for that patient. Make it applicable to the patient's condition and the (differential) diagnoses you've made. It is of little value just to tell the patient to call back if they have chest pain if their presenting complaint is of a neurological aetiology. How you provide a safety net for your patient is important: engage the patient, their family members, care line pendant provider, nurse or carer to ensure there is an awareness and expectation. Specify information or resources used to signpost the patient about their condition. Remember that worsening care advice and safety netting are only necessary because diseases are not always typical, clinicians do not always get it right first time and healthcare is rarely completely predictable or deterministic.

Conclusion

In this chapter, we have discussed the importance of sharing decisions and appreciating that paramedic practice can be very isolated in certain practice settings. The decision making in practice is not always straightforward; a decision might seem wholly wrong and unreasonable to one clinician, whereas to another it might seem completely sensible. The undifferentiated and unpredictable patient cohorts we see mean that we need to think dynamically, with a willingness to adapt the plan to suit the needs of the situation.

We have discussed experience and the importance of filling your years with reflection and learning. Also, the risks of over-testing and how ambulance services are quite vulnerable without the vast choice of tests available elsewhere. You are able to make your decisions defensible and reasonable by considering the needs of the patient in front of you. By now, you should be beginning to think more dynamically about your decisions and how best to serve the communities you work in by making choices that will not only benefit the patient in front of you, but also the next ones you will see too.

Reflective Exercises

1. Consider Mo from the start of the chapter. Is there anything that could've been done differently, and anything you would have done to help manage the risk here?
2. How does your current approach to documentation align with the published standards? Write a real or fictional case study where discharge is involved. After it is written, review it against the regulatory or practice standards. Is it sufficiently detailed and contemporaneous? Does it include relevant safety netting, referencing appropriate resource tools for self-help and relevant worsening care advice?
3. Aside from the ones listed – what other 'dangerous diagnoses' and red flags can you think of that are frequently given to patients in practice without due consideration for the other, more subtle, ones?
4. Think about the value of feedback. How would finding out that you were wrong about a diagnosis make you feel and how could this affect your practice? How could you better learn from feedback?

Chapter 8

Case-based Discussion (Case Studies, Reflection, Action Learning)

Andy Collen, Si Robinson, Kieren Pugh and Sean Teed

Introduction

This chapter looks at a series of seven case studies typical in paramedic practice settings. Each of these has very clear decision points, which can be reflected upon and linked to the concepts discussed throughout this book. The cases are intended to be high-level examples and they intentionally lack some of the details that might be seen in practice. As with all written case studies, there is none of the sensory clues we usually have access to in order to enrich the context of our encounters with patients or clients (sights, smells etc.). Despite this, the narrower dimension of written examples can be imagined in real-life practice settings, and can serve to begin prompting the use of 'decision point management' – those forks in the road upon which subsequent decisions rely.

The cases may not provide exhaustive information on every possible aspect of the scenario, and you should use any gaps you find as an opportunity to expand on the story and make further enquiry. This will provide even more opportunity to develop your skills and broaden your thinking beyond what you can see or read.

Importantly, the case studies use a 'before and after' layout, highlighting the biases and fogs, and have some obviously intuitive outcomes which may, or may not, be correct. Remember, the most important aspect is the process you follow to achieve the answer – not the answer itself, as this may cause hindsight bias as a result.

Please note – all the case studies use standard medical clerking headings/abbreviations:

- HPC: History of presenting complaint
- PMH: Previous medical (and/or surgical) history
- Allergies: Including medicines and foods
- DH: Drug history – prescribed and over-the-counter medicines taken
- SH: Social history (how they live)
- SE: System evaluation (sometimes called 'review of systems') – asks the patient or client about symptoms organized by system, i.e. headaches

- OE: On examination – findings of physical assessments
- IMP: Impression – the working diagnosis
- Plan: Onward plan of care.

Case Study 1: 32-year-old Female with a Headache

Background

You are working on a single response unit. It is a Saturday night shift at midnight, and you have already attended five calls since you started your shift at 19:00. It is your second night of your set of shifts. You are called to a 32-year-old female with a headache and hyperventilation. On arrival, you find your patient conscious and talking but extremely anxious. She is accompanied by her partner, who is eager to get the all clear so they can continue their evening.

- HPC: Patient has been out this evening and has consumed several glasses of wine and spirits (around 8 units of alcohol), she has returned home earlier than planned due to feeling unwell. Has vomited once and since felt better. An hour later, the patient was having intercourse when the onset of headache occurred. Her partner called 911 when she started to hyperventilate and he became worried about her breathing.
- PMH: Migraine, Dysmenorrhea.
- Allergies: None.
- DH: Rizatriptan, oral contraceptive pill (OCP), tranexamic acid (TXA).
- SH: Lives alone.
- SE: Patient complains of generalized headache, atypical prodrome for migraine (no aura). Denies chest pain. All other review-of-systems responses are unremarkable.
- Vital sign and clinical observations all within normal limits.
- IMP: Migraine headache and hyperventilation due to emotional factors.
- Plan: Leave at home in the care of partner.

Potential Outcome for This Patient with Poor Decision Making

Intuitive Responses

This presentation carries a range of risks, and led to a decision being made entirely intuitively. Perhaps the clinician was thinking: 'This must be a migraine. She has been drinking, and this has made her emotional and panicky. The hyperventilation is emotional in origin and can be managed with coaching'. This only describes 'what' that they are seeing or perceiving. There is no consideration of 'why'. Why, for example, must the hyperventilation have been caused by emotional factors? Hyperventilation may be emotional in origin, but could also be linked to sinister metabolic disturbance.

Migraine sufferers may also have inter-cranial bleeds, and are at higher risk of mortality due to history of primary headaches being incorrectly attributed to acute secondary headache. Coital headaches are usually self-limiting and may not have accompanying focal neurology.

Biases and Fallacies

Review the section on 'Human Fallibility and Biased Thinking' in Chapter 3 to find the biases used in the example.

- **Association bias** – Young females are prone to hyperventilation and anxiety (a picture of a young female hyperventilating is common).
- **Availability bias** – 'Emotional patient' must mean hyperventilation is emotional in origin.

What other biases and fallacies may be involved with this case?

Human Factors

- Saturday night shift (fatigue, workload, staffing levels etc.)
- Lone working
- Work intensity (number of incidents attended already)
- Tiredness
- Lack of team or other colleague to share ideas with.

What other human factors may be involved with this case?

The Worst Outcome for This Patient with Poor Decision Making

The decision is made to leave the patient at home with her boyfriend. No worsening care advice is documented, and no safety netting is provided. In the early hours, the patient becomes more sleepy and so is put to bed by her boyfriend. Her ICP rises (due to an undiagnosed intracranial bleed) and causes increasing coma, but this is unmonitored. The next morning, her boyfriend is unable to wake her and calls 911, who provide pre-arrival CPR instruction. An ambulance attends and the crew are unable to resuscitate the patient despite an extended period of ALS. Following application of all available interventions, the decision is taken to cease resuscitation (using appropriate decision-making process to ensure all reversible causes are addressed).

Potential Outcome for This Patient with Good Decision Making

Information Processing (Critical Analysis of Data and Information)

- History of migraine may be a fog – atypical presentation. If the patient didn't have a history of migraine, would you consider the presentation as a primary or secondary headache?

- Consideration of health history, including drug history.
- Coital headache (this onset of which may be mid-coital) – not always sinister, but sinister aspects need to be ruled out.
- Alcohol consumption may mask true level of consciousness.
- Poor historian – patient has consumed alcohol.
- Patient's boyfriend may not be worried as he wishes to continue with his evening.

Professional Insights

- I do not have the neurological assessment skills or diagnostics to rule out sinister pathology (*I know what I don't know*).
- I do not know enough about headaches and patients with migraine.
- I know the key differential diagnoses for headache but cannot definitively rule in/out.

Hypotheses/Differential Diagnoses (With Positive Features –!)

- Meningitis
- **Encephalitis**
- Sub-arachnoid haemorrhage**!**
- Head injury
- Sinusitis
- Tropical illness (e.g., malaria)
- Pre-eclampsia**!** (vomiting – unknown if patient is pregnant)
- Hypertensive crisis
- Migraine**!**
- Coital headache**!**
- Trigeminal neuralgia
- Glaucoma

Deductive Reasoning

- This patient may need further assessment and imaging (MRI/CT) based on the likely differential diagnoses.
- I have reached my capability line (see Chapter 5) and cannot reach a definitive diagnosis.
- I have both insufficient skills and diagnostic equipment to rule out sinister pathology.

- The only solution is to refer this patient on for further assessment.

Ethical Considerations

- Vulnerability – intoxication and in care of boyfriend (consideration should be given to the relationship status, i.e., have they just met or are they in a stable, long-term relationship?)
- Non-maleficence – prevent harm coming to patient.
- Justice – has the patient received the best care/service they deserve?

Professional Issues

- Practising to your scope of practice and level of competency.
- Advocating for your patient.

The Best Outcome Using Good Decision-making Processes

This patient has a sudden onset headache and has several other issues, which make it impossible to make a definitive diagnosis in this setting. A key decision as to whether to make a clinical diagnosis or refer for imaging is an intrinsic consideration of decision making in urgent and emergency care.

The patient was therefore sent to the Emergency Department immediately and deteriorated in the ambulance en-route to the hospital. On arrival, the crew were met by a team and the patient was intubated and had a CT scan. She was found to have an intracranial bleed. The plan of care was conservative treatment, and she was woken on Day 3. She was discharged from hospital around a week later with no neurological deficit.

Decision Making: Assessment and Key Learning Points

Primary headaches (spontaneous in nature, such as generalized headaches) are common, and can be mistaken for secondary headaches (resulting from disease, such as a brain tumour) where the causation isn't obvious. The decision making in this case was as much about logical information processing than achieving diagnostic certainty. It was clear early on that to leave the patient at home was to take a very significant risk, and in the 'before' case led to a very poor outcome. Even if the decision had been to leave the patient at home, the decision point management was very weak in the 'before' part of the case study and there was no safety netting provided. This case highlights the risks of making intuitive decisions, which can be influenced by associative biases, and in a setting that may introduce additional risks from human factors (i.e., fatigue). Stepping back and assessing the quality of the information, and processing it in a step-wise way before testing each hypothesis, will lead to an end point. That end point may not be a diagnosis, but may be the point where you reach the limit of your capability, suggesting the need to refer on to hospital. The decision to say you cannot reach a diagnosis and need to refer on may affect how we feel (bruised pride, frustration). Reaching such a decision requires good levels of professional insight and self-confidence. Remembering that the patient is paramount (safety, outcomes, justice) and striving to learn from our experiences are key aspects of professional practice.

Case Study 2: 45-year-old Male with Productive Cough and Chest Pain

Background

You are working on an ambulance with a junior colleague and have been on duty since 08:00. It been a quiet start to the shift, and at 08:17 you receive a 911 call to a 45-year-old male with a cough and chest pain.

The patient is being nagged by his partner, who is claiming he is 'putting it on' and has 'man-flu'. She was ill last week, and he didn't care when she was feeling poorly. The partner continually interrupts the encounter between you and patient.

- HPC: 5/7 history of productive cough with fever, complaining of feeling weak and suffering 'aches and pains'. Over past 24 hours, coughing frequency has increased and he is finding it harder to clear his throat. He now has pains across chest – described as 'muscular' and 'aching'.
- PMH: Hypertension (recent diagnosis).
- Allergies: NKDA.
- DH: ACE inhibitor.
- SH: Lives with girlfriend. Unemployed.
- SE: Denies headache or other neurological signs or symptoms. C/O increased sputum production and expectoration. C/O pain across chest – patient generalizes area affected across whole chest. Pain worse when coughing.
- OE: Hypertensive; HR 84 and regular; BG 5.6 mmol/L; Temp 38.0°C.
- IMP: Chest infection. Chest pain muscular and caused by coughing.
- Plan: Suggest to be seen at a walk in clinic or see GP later that morning for antibiotics. Remain in care of partner.

Potential Outcome for This Patient with Poor Decision Making

Intuitive Responses

There are obvious signs of a chest infection, and this is probably a correct diagnosis in isolation, but remember that patients can have two acute illnesses at the same time. The crew may have been thinking: 'Clearly, the patient has a chest infection and is too young to be having a heart attack. Therefore, the chest pain can be accounted for due to the many days of constant coughing.'

This patient should see his GP to get some antibiotics. We can leave him at home with his girlfriend.

Biases and Fallacies

Review the section on 'Human Fallibility and Biased Thinking' in Chapter 3 to find the biases used in the example.

- **Stereotyping** – Men don't tolerate minor health problems well. He probably called 911 because he was fed up with being ill.
- **Association bias** – Associating the productive cough, fever and chest pain with a simple diagnosis. The symptoms lend themselves to the diagnosis.
- **Availability bias** – Experience may lead to a recall of more middle-aged men with chest infections than heart attacks. The availability and association biases have conspired to prevent effective inquiry into the true cause and nature of the chest pain.

What other biases and fallacies may be involved with this case?

Human Factors

- **Distractions and interruptions** – the patient's partner was being disruptive and dismissive.
- **Human error** – the crew missed the other cause of the chest pain.
- **Poor information processing** – the chest pain being muscular was not processed effectively.
- **Vigilance** – the crew did not diligently ensure the patient was safe and used their intuition to drive their plan.

What other human factors may be involved with this case?

A Poor Outcome for This Patient with Poor Decision Making

The diagnosis given of chest infection was correct, but unrelated to this illness this patient also suffered a myocardial infarction, causing chest pain, weakness and feeling ill. The true retrosternal chest pain was masked by the muscular pains and the patient's other symptoms.

After being discharged from the paramedics' care, the patient went back to bed and rested for about 90 minutes and then rose to go to the toilet. At this point he collapsed to the floor, which was witnessed by his partner. She commenced CPR and called 911, receiving pre-arrival advice. A crew arrived in around 7 minutes and found the patient to have a pulse but unconscious. Upon moving to the vehicle, the patient re-arrested and was given advanced life support before gaining ROSC again. He was taken to hospital and underwent primary percutaneous coronary intervention (pPCI) to clear his occluded coronary artery. He went on to make a good recovery.

Potential Outcome for This Patient with Good Decision Making

Information Processing (Critical Analysis of Data and Information)

- Chest pain is always sinister and needs investigating (i.e., ECG).
- In the presence of other disease processes, other signs and symptoms may lose their typical nature or quality. In this case, the chest pain becoming masked by the muscular discomfort. The weakness and feeling of illness were attributed solely to an infection.
- There was no attempt to find out 'why' the patient had chest pain – the clinicians only focused on the 'what'.
- Innate egocentrism – the clinicians believed they were correct, so thought their decision was correct without questioning it.

Professional Insights

- A potential lack of understanding of own limitations.
- Use of experience and intuition without personal challenge.

Hypotheses/Differential Diagnoses (With Positive Features –!)

- Acute coronary syndrome (ACS)**!**
- Dissecting thoracic aneurysm**!**
- Pericarditis/myocarditis**!**
- Acute congestive cardiac failure
- Pulmonary embolus**!**
- Acute pancreatitis
- Oesophageal rupture
- Pneumonia/lower respiratory tract infection.

Deductive Reasoning

- This patient has chest pain as well as other symptoms indicative of bacterial or viral illness.
- The patient has problems I cannot visualize and so needs diagnostic tests.
- I can do some diagnostic tests, such as ECG, but I cannot access all of the tests I need in the community.
- My working diagnosis does not rule out sinister causes for chest pain – it only rules in a chest infection.

- Therefore, this patient has undifferentiated acute chest pain and should attend hospital for repeat ECG and troponin tests.
- I have reached my capability line (see Chapter 5) and cannot reach a definitive diagnosis.
- The safe and logical decision is to convey this patient to an Emergency Department.

Ethical Considerations

- This patient did not get just levels of care – his needs were not addressed due to poor decision making and lack of systematic assessment.
- This case was not approached in a beneficent way. The care was not applied in the patient's best interest or on the basis of providing sufficient information for the patient to be informed about their health needs.

Professional Issues

In this case, several CPCF standards may have not been applied:

1. Practise safely, competently, compassionately, and ethically, and be accountable for their competence to patients, the regulator, the employer, the profession, and the public.

2. Attain, maintain, and demonstrate the appropriate competencies (knowledge, skills, and attitudes) to practise safely and provide patient-centred care.

3. Demonstrate behaviours that uphold the public's trust in the profession.

There was a lack of competency in the way the patient was managed, and it could be argued that patient-centred care was not provided.

The Best Outcome Using Good Decision-making Processes

This patient suffered a myocardial infarction about an hour prior to calling the ambulance for his worsening infective symptoms. When the ambulance crew arrived, they initially focused on the chest pain, rather than the fever or other infective signs and symptoms (mindful of the risk of severe sepsis, of course). They completed an initial ECG, which showed extensive ST segment elevation indicating an anterior infarct. They completed the STEMI care bundle (aspirin, nitrates, analgesia), and took the patient directly to the pPCI centre following a discussion with the team at the hospital. The clot was resolved successfully, and at no point did the patient go into cardiac arrest. After the pPCI was completed, the patient was treated for a severe chest infection alongside his cardiac aftercare.

Decision-making Assessment and Key Learning Points

While such scenarios are rare, they underpin the importance of avoiding the risk of dismissing other possibilities simply because they are rare. We have discussed previously the danger of using terms such as: 'If it looks like a duck and sounds like a duck, it's probably is a duck'. It could be argued that the chest infection looked and sounded like a duck, but where the two diseases (chest infection and MI) are blended, it becomes a different animal that is extremely rare and doesn't look like anything seen before.

In this case, the outcome didn't change, and the additional 90-minute delay between the initial 911 call and the eventual collapse had a minimal impact on the long-term outcome, but that is not the point. How many times are bullets dodged without our knowledge, and how many times are we correct or incorrect without knowing?

Case Study 3: 78-year-old Female Fallen with a Minor Head Injury and Taking Anticoagulant Therapy

Background

You are working in the emergency department in the fast track (Pod) area with the physicians in the department and your parter who just started working as a paramedic in the ED. Triage has sent an older client who fell at home that morning to your Pod for treatment and has prioritized them as a CTAS (Canadian Triage Acuity Score) 4. Her sister is with her and is worried about this morning's fall. Georgie is a 79-year-old woman who, for her age, is in very good health. There are many admitted patients still waiting in the ED for beds to free up on the floor. The hope is that Georgie can be treated for her scalp laceration and discharged fairly quickly to help with the emergency department wait times. You are very keen to demonstrate your wound care competencies and contribute to the positive workflow through the ED.

- HPC: Slipped from her chair while stretching to put something on a nearby table and hit her head on the corner of an adjacent piece of furniture. The wound on her head has bled profusely and is being managed with a tea-towel and cold compress from her sister.
- PMH: Atrial fibrillation.
- Allergies: Elastoplast.
- DH: Apixaban.
- SH: Lives with sister in an independent living setting. No other family. Has meals on wheels and is able to perform here ADLs with no issues.
- SE: The patient says she feels rather silly falling out of her chair as she did. She is worried about the blood staining the carpet. She denies headache or any other injuries, but does admit that she caught her head with quite some force. No nausea or vomiting. Able to mobilize with assistance.
- OE: Neurological exam unremarkable (cranial nerve assessment, PERRLA, Romberg's test, PNS gross movement, 'Time Up and Go'). GCS 15 – no loss of consciousness. 5 cm laceration to vertex, bleeding freely. Large haematoma forming. All other systems/observations unremarkable or normal for patient (AF).

- IMP: Minor fall in the home with head wound/injury. Not on Warfarin, so safe to treat at home.
- Plan: Close wound with hair apposition technique (HAT). Discharge into care of sister. Return to ED if signs of head injury or concussion develop.

Potential Outcome for This Patient with Poor Decision Making

Intuitive Responses

'The main issue the EDP (Emergency Department Physician) wants me to focus on is the head wound, so that the EDP can bring more patients into the fast track area. I am anxious to demonstrate my wound care skills and keen to also improve ED flow.'

The paramedic in this case has discounted the fall as being sinister and is instead focusing on closing the wound, safe in the knowledge that the patient is not on warfarin and so is not at risk of a bleed. There is a presumption that the head wound is the only issue, and the fall has already been deemed minor. Logically, the EDP cannot possibly know the magnitude of the fall based on a triage chart / note alone. The lack of any wider context has further served to blinker the attending paramedic, and these factors are conspiring to promote a poorly conceived intuitive response. Moreover, the well-established heuristic knowledge about the link between Warfarin and head injuries in older patients, and the lack of knowledge and awareness of the novel (newer) anticoagulant drugs (NOACs), further prevents structured enquiry.

Biases and Fallacies

Review the section on 'Human Fallibility and Biased Thinking' in Chapter 3 to find the biases used in the example.

- **Confirmation bias** – This patient was triaged as a CTAS 4 (medium/lower acuity) and 'just requiring repair of laceration' by another professional who also did not recognize the anticoagulant.
- **Authority bias** – Unconditional belief in what the EDP said about the patient's needs.
- **Availability bias** – There was an understanding of Warfarin in context to head injury, and the absence of that medicine provided a basis to make the wrong decision because the knowledge was available (remember, we often don't know what we don't know).

What other biases and fallacies may be involved with this case?

Human Factors

- **Environment** – ED is overcrowded with admitted patients and attempts to improve flow of new patients through the ED.
- **Team** – being on placement with a different group of staff and professional groups.

- **Adverse event** – the error has led to harm to the patient.
- **Education and training** – did the paramedic have sufficient training?

What other human factors may be involved with this case?

A Poor Outcome for This Patient with Poor Decision Making

The patient and her sister were delighted with the care they received at the time. The patient was made comfortable in a treatment and the head wound attended to. The wound was thoroughly cleaned and closed with tissue adhesive and hair giving a very good aesthetic result. The haematoma was still present but not getting worse and a further cold compress was applied. Oral analgesia was given, and the patient received head injury advice, including what to do if she felt ill in due course.

Later that afternoon, the patient started complaining of headache and nausea, and soon after vomited twice. Her sister noticed that she was unsteady and appeared a little confused.

Meanwhile, the patient has started to lose consciousness and her sister calls 911. A crew arrive and take the patient to hospital where an extradural haemorrhage is noted. The patient is actively treated and recovers from the bleed and undergoes a period of rehabilitation before being discharged into a residential home, along with her sister.

The outcome for this patient is unlikely to have changed had the red flag been noted sooner. The outcome could easily have been that the patient died quickly from a more rapidly developing bleed, and similarly a slower bleed could have led to coma during sleep that night. There are several factors relating to this case, but the most significant root cause is the lack of knowledge of common prescribing in older patients with AF. Novel anticoagulants (NOACs) are more commonly used, and have a wider range of drug names such as Apixaban, Dabigatran Etexilate, Edoxaban and Rivaroxaban, which need to be understood. In the past, Warfarin was most commonly used and became a heuristically embedded, universally understood risk factor.

Potential Outcome for This Patient with Good Decision Making

Information Processing (Critical Analysis of Data and Information)

- Older patient fallen – Why did she fall? Have all the red flags associated with older patients falling been considered?
- History of head injury – In older patients, the index of suspicion is far higher for brain injury, even if they are not symptomatic at the time.
- History of atrial fibrillation – Why can I not see an anticoagulant on her prescription?
- Drug history reviewed but not understood – Patient has AF, but anticoagulant (warfarin) not seen (see, 'Where's the bomb' in Chapter 5).

- Large developing haematoma at wound site – Freely bleeding wound and a developing haematoma may suggest anticoagulant use. Recheck the medicines!

Professional Insights

- I am confident and competent to manage the wound, but may lack the insight to assess my own ability to manage wounds in older or complex patients.
- I don't know every common medicine used in primary care.
- The clinician may have thought: '.I know most of the policies and clinical practice guidelines on wound closure.'
- Innate self-validation – 'It's true because I have always believed it'; 'Warfarin is the most common anticoagulant and the only one I know. So it may be the only one.'

Hypotheses/Differential Diagnoses (With Positive Features –!)

- Intracranial bleed secondary to trauma**!** (based on risk factors)
- Skull fracture
- Minor scalp wound**!**
- Haematoma to scalp**!**
- Associated causes of fall**!**

Deductive Reasoning

- This patient has a large scalp wound and developing haematoma.
- She is an older patient, but essentially well.
- I can manage her wound, and should do so.
- She has suffered a blow to the head but appears neurologically intact.
- She has AF. Is she taking medicines to prevent clotting?
- There are medicines in her prescription that I don't recognize – I will check.
- Apixaban is an anticoagulant.
- This patient has a scalp wound with a potential underlying brain injury.

Ethical Considerations

In this case, the paramedic was very confident about how to manage the wound and became overly focused on this to the exclusion of the holistic needs of the patient. It is important to see patients as paramount, and never as a means to an end. The keenness to apply the new wound care skills could be seen as using the patient as a means to an end. It is important to approach patients based on their needs in relation to their illness or injury, rather than your own professional development and practice.

Professional Issues

Clinicians must ensure that they are competent to practise and must be able to demonstrate that patients are not at risk where there is a gap in knowledge or skill.

The paramedic was unaware of the gaps in their knowledge, which led to an overall lack of competence in addressing the patient's needs. This in itself is not an issue, as there is always the option to defer to a colleague for support and to share decisions. This requires a high level of professional insight, though, as well as the ability to assess one's own level of competency. It is far better to suffer a small dent in your pride than to harm a patient.

The Best Outcome Using Good Decision-making Processes

Using a deductive process that builds hypotheses on critically assessed information allows certain factors to be tested and challenged. The key red flag relating to anticoagulant therapy has been identified and the patient is now taken to the emergency department. Early treatment is conservative, and the patient is monitored for several hours, and the same deterioration is noted in the emergency department. The scenario from here plays out in exactly the same way, with the patient making a good recovery.

Decision-making Assessment and Key Learning Points

This case highlights the importance of professional insight and ensuring that any gaps in knowledge do not lead to risk of harm to patients. The deductive process, using logical arguments based on the information present, highlighted very quickly a link between the patient's condition, their acute problem, and their drug history (or apparent lack of drug history). Just because something you expect isn't there, doesn't mean it doesn't exist. A patient with a freely bleeding wound and who has AF is very likely to be on an anticoagulant, and that medicine may be unfamiliar to you. How often do we look at a patient's list of medicines – particularly in the older patient where the list may be very long – and ignore items that are not familiar? Where a condition such as AF exists, the clinician should draw on the deductive process to resolve the likely treatment regime that is supported by evidence and best practice. Remember the story from Rosenorn-Langg – airport security staff do not simply allow bags to pass through the x-ray scanner saying 'no bomb, no bomb, no, bomb', instead they ask themselves 'where's the bomb?' – 'actively looking', rather than 'not seeing' (Rosenorn-Langg, 2014, p. 1).

Case Study 4: 29-year-old Female with Respiratory Illness

Background

You are working on a fixed-wing air ambulance and are called to a busy northern community clinic on a Thursday afternoon. It has been a steady day and youand your partner have flown most of the day and have seen a range of clients with minor illnesses and injuries throughout the day. At about 20:00 you arrive at the clinic to see the next patient. The patient and her partner meet you to in the exam room. The client is a 29-year-old female with a 5-day history of cough and fever. This is her third clinic visit over the past two days. She has been seen by an NP and an ambulance crew previously, who have all suggested a self-limiting viral illness.

- HPC: 5/7 history of worsening productive cough and increasing weakness.
- PMH: Appendicectomy aged 13. Three children, all delivered by C-section.
- Allergies: NKDA.
- DH: Oral contraceptive pill.
- SH: Lives with husband and three children. Works part time for the local authority housing team.
- SE: Complains of feeling awful. Says she 'feels like she is dying'. She appears panicky and her partner reports feeling frustrated that she is still ill, and his parents are having to look after the kids. Wants to know why she is still ill and not getting better. Patient complains of feeling shivery and is coughing +++. (No further systems history reviewed as focus on viral illness affecting chest.)
- OE: HR 118 bpm; RR 22; BP 88/45 mmHg; SpO_2 94%; Temp 38.2°C. Some adventitious chest sounds on auscultation but hard to discern as patient coughing.
- IMP: Based on previous encounters, which included a GP virtual consult, agree that this is likely to be a viral illness that will resolve with self-care.
- Plan: Discharge with advice to use acetaminophen PRN to manage fever. Aim to maintain hydration by taking clear fluids (water, dilute fruit juice) regularly.

Potential Outcome for This Patient with Poor Decision Making

Intuitive Responses

She has been seen by her NP and a GP virtually who has told her what is wrong, and I am worried about looking foolish if I disagree with the GP and NP. I do not want to contradict a senior clinician. The ambulance crew didn't find anything either presumably, as she wasn't taken to hospital. The history and symptoms still fit with the diagnosis, and the increased heart and respiratory rate are probably because she is tired and anxious. It all seems to fit, and she can always come back if she doesn't get better.

Biases and Fallacies

Review the section on 'Human Fallibility and Biased Thinking' in Chapter 3 to find the biases used in the example.

- **Authority bias** – Concern about contradicting the opinion of the GP and NP because they are senior healthcare professionals.

- **Groupthink** – In this case, the paramedic, the ambulance crew, the NP and the GP all fall into a common belief that the patient had a self-limiting viral illness. Groupthink can occur where information is passed around, such as in this case, and leads to a lack of challenge from each recipient.
- **Neglect of probability** – Common things happen commonly, and rare things happen rarely – but they still happen. Considering probability is important.

What other biases and fallacies may be involved with this case?

Human Factors

- **Stressors of flight** – including noise, vibration, temperature and pressure changes which contribute to poor decision making.
- **Information processing** – Lack of critical analysis of the physiological impact of the patient's condition. The observations were clearly abnormal, but were considered in the context of an existing diagnosis presumed to be correct.
- **Latent error** – The NP, GP and the previously attending ambulance crew all potentially made an error in judging the patient's condition (although the patient may have presented with milder or more subtle signs earlier).
- **Vigilance** – The nature of work in certain clinical settings, particularly where another clinician with higher authority has already made a diagnosis, may lead to sense of false security leading to potentially missing very unwell patients.

What other human factors may be involved with this case?

A Poor Outcome for This Patient with Poor Decision Making

The patient left the consulting room and walked back to the waiting room while her husband went to collect the car because she felt she couldn't walk far to it. After her husband left the waiting room, the patient passes out and falls to the floor. The receptionist notices this and goes over to the patient to find her unrousable and without a detectable pulse. She shouts for help while commencing CPR. Staff leave their consulting room to attend to the patient and an ambulance is called. The combined efforts of the ambulance paramedics and UCC staff lead to a return of spontaneous circulation, and the patient is stabilized and taken to the local hospital. Her observations are now that of a critically unwell patient, and she is carefully intubated and transferred to ITU. She requires inotropic support, as well as other interventions, but sadly on Day 2 it becomes clear that overwhelming sepsis has already caused irreversible organ damage, and the patient goes into cardiac arrest. Despite the best efforts of the team, the resuscitation attempt is terminated after 90 minutes.

Potential Outcome for This Patient with Good Decision Making

Information Processing (Critical Analysis of Data and Information)

- History of illness that is not improving and seems to be getting worse.
- The patient is using classic terminology associated with sepsis ('I think I am dying').
- Why did the GP think this was a viral illness, and were they correct? I should challenge their findings.
- Why did the ambulance crew also think this was a viral illness, and what made them confirm the GP's diagnosis?
- The patient's observations are outside normal ranges suggesting a systemic effect from the illness.
- Do I have enough information to make a decision? I need to expand my review of systems (SE) to include additional questions about passing urine, which would have elicited that she hasn't urinated in over 8 hours. What is her NEWS score and what are the individual elements, such as the blood pressure?

Professional Insights

- Have I approached this patient correctly and not dismissed their needs because they have already seen another healthcare professional?
- Do I have the necessary skills to assess this patient in this practice setting, and does my scope of practice extend to the nature of the condition presenting?
- Am I prepared to ask for assistance in this case?
- Am I prepared to question and/or contradict an NP's or GP's diagnosis?

Hypotheses/Differential Diagnoses (With Positive Features –!)

The following are secondary to the presence of severe sepsis as the chief complaint, and may be considered as the focus of the infection:

- Upper respiratory tract infection
- Acute bronchitis**!**
- Pneumonia**!**
- Pulmonary embolism
- Bronchiectasis
- Pleurisy.

Deductive Reasoning

- This patient has an infective illness that is affecting her physiology and appears therefore to be systemic.
- This systemic infection appears to be affecting her perfusion (high NEWS score and not passing urine).
- The patient is severely septic. This patient should be transported to hospital and potentially tertiary care and consider EGT.

Ethical Considerations

- **Non-maleficence** – It is vital to prevent harm coming to the patient, and this extends to ensuring diseases are identified and their progression minimized.
- **Justice** – The patient has had three healthcare encounters and yet has not been given the correct care.

Professional Issues

In this case, there was a lack of appreciation of the needs of the patient, and the lack of structured decision making placed the patient in jeopardy. It is reasonable to consider the possibility that had the patient self-presented to the urgent care centre without first seeing other healthcare professionals/services, a more thorough assessment may have taken place.

The Best Outcome Using Good Decision-making Processes

The patient presented to the urgent care centre and was called through by the paramedic. When the patient mentioned the previous diagnosis given by the GP, which was subsequently confirmed by the ambulance crew, the paramedic makes it clear to the patient that they would assess her thoroughly and objectively and that she was correct to attend this afternoon. It quickly becomes apparent that despite the vital signs and the previous diagnosis given, this patient has severe sepsis. She is gravely ill, but is currently compensating well. The patient is screened using an evidence informed screening tool, and transport to a higher level of care is arranged. An air ambulance arrives within 10 minutes and the patient receives early goal directed therapy and is flown to hospital. In flight, she receives IV antibiotics and is transferred to ICU. She remains unstable for the first 24 hours, but eventually improves and recovers. She is discharged several weeks later and has damage to her kidneys, but is grateful to be alive. The ICU consultant stated upon her discharge how close to death she had been at one point.

Decision-making Assessment and Key Learning Points

On some occasions, logical deduction drives the type of management rather than the final diagnosis. This patient's overall condition raised alarm in the paramedic in the 'best outcome' section, and this intuition appropriately drove hypotheses, which in turn led to screening the patient against known parameters (the sepsis tool). While a respiratory illness was most likely, the final diagnosis was not made. In the case of severe sepsis, it is more important to resuscitate than to find the type or focus of the infection, as antibiotic therapy may be given empirically rather than waiting for microbiology tests to confirm the bug causing the infection. More importantly is the need to ensure that a decision is made, and that previous decisions are not adopted without your own enquiry. This case shows how easy it can be to write off a patient with very marked features of disease processes – both in terms of signs and symptoms, and changes to their physiology – just because another clinician has given a diagnosis. If the paramedic had not been aware of the previous assessments or the 911 call that the ambulance crew attended, would they have thought differently?

Case Study 5: 36-year-old Female with Abdominal Pain

Background

You are working in a single response unit as a community care paramedic on a Sunday night shift in early summer. At about midnight, you receive a 911 call to a female complaining of abdominal pain. The call has originated as a non-urgent transport call, which has been pushed to 911 response due to the responses to the triage questions.

On arrival, you are taken to the patient, who is lying on the sofa watching television. She complains of lower abdominal discomfort.

- HPC: 3/7 history of 'gripey' pain. Non-radiating. No fever. Patient states she is 'fed up with the pain' and wants to feel better.
- PMH: Two recent terminations of pregnancy (both in the last 12 months). Learning disability. Mild asthma.
- Allergies: NKDA.
- DH: None.
- SH: Lives with partner. Works part-time in local shop. Has a support worker who assists with certain aspects of her life.
- SE: Complains of pain across lower abdomen. Bowels open normally and no concerns regarding 'water works'.

  Nauseated. Vomited x 1. No diarrhoea.

  Denies headache, chest pain and breathing problems. All other systems reviewed are negative to symptoms.

  Denies pregnancy and denies sexual activity.
- OE: HR 105; RR 16; BP 105/65 mmHg; SpO_2 98%; Pain score 6/10.

  Abdomen soft. Tender to light palpation in LLQ and RLQ.

- IMP: Abdominal pain in a patient of child-bearing age with a recent history of termination of pregnancy.
- Plan: Seek consent to undertake urinalysis and confirm findings (**bHCG** +ve. Blood ++).

Potential Outcome for This Patient with Poor Decision Making

Intuitive Responses

This patient has abdominal pain, and I know that if I try for a diagnosis, I am likely to be wrong. (According to Simon et al., 2005, 50% of initial diagnoses for abdominal pain are wrong.) The patient may not fully understand the questions I am asking about being pregnant or the true meaning of sexual activity due to her learning difficulty. I am also concerned about her potential vulnerability and the history of multiple terminations. I am going ask the patient for a urine sample to test for a potential urinary tract infection, but also to ensure she is not pregnant.

Biases and Fallacies

Review the section on 'Human Fallibility and Biased Thinking' in Chapter 3 to find the biases used in the example.

- **False causality** – Assumption that a patient with learning disability is unaware of her own sexual health. She may be aware but unable to express this in terms understood by those not known to the patient.
- **Conjunction** – Linking the cause of a potential unknown pregnancy to the patient's competency. The cause of the abdominal pain is an undetected ectopic pregnancy, not the patient's learning disability.
- **Feature-positive effect** – This has been avoided in this case. Commonly, things that cannot be seen are ignored, and in this case the potential issue has been identified and searched for.

What other biases and fallacies may be involved with this case?

Human Factors

- **Skills gap** – Lack of knowledge of learning disabilities.
- **Communication** – Loss of opportunity to ask the patient to express herself in her own terms.

What other human factors may be involved with this case?

Actual Outcome for This Patient with Poor Decision Making

The decision making in this case was technically very good. The possibility of being unaware of a pregnancy and linking this to the cause of abdominal pain was well founded through logical thought process and critical analysis of the information. Linked to this was the insight into the limitations of one's own practice.

There are some limitations with the approach to the patient's learning disability, and this has skewed the decision-making process due to biases and a lack of appreciation of the patient's functional ability.

Overall, this case describes good decision-making process and a good outcome. This scenario could have turned out very differently had the paramedic not applied a logical approach to the problem and simply trusted the patient. The differential diagnoses for a young female who is not pregnant has very few, if any, immediately sinister pathologies, and therefore missing the pregnancy (which in this case was ectopic) would represent a potentially life-threatening problem.

Actual Outcome for This Patient with Good Decision Making

Information Processing (Critical Analysis of Data and Information)

- History of abdominal pain – Clinical diagnoses may be wrong in 50% of cases. Usually need follow up in secondary care. Where sinister conditions can be ruled out, follow up may be done more routinely.
- Learning disability – The patient functions well with minimal support in the community, but may not be able to express themselves, and this makes their history harder to elicit.
- Previous history of elective termination of pregnancy – What were the circumstances, and do these represent a safeguarding issue? (Consider referral.)
- Abdomen tender.
- Pregnancy test positive.
- Reliability of urinalysis.

Professional Insights

- I am not confident to rule out sinister pathology in a patient with a learning disability, as I do not understand it sufficiently.
- I may not be able to communicate as effectively with this patient and I need to be careful in how I ask them to undertake a urine test to check for pregnancy.

Hypotheses/Differential Diagnoses (With Positive Features –!)

- Appendicitis**!**
- Pelvic inflammatory disease**!**

- Pregnancy!
- Ectopic pregnancy!
- Hernia!
- Diverticulitis!
- Bowel obstruction!
- UTI
- Pyelonephritis
- Ruptured ovarian cyst!
- Bowel perforation
- Inflammatory bowel disease!

Deductive Reasoning

- This patient has a history of abdominal pain.
- Abdominal pain is very challenging to definitively diagnose in the community unless sinister features can be excluded.
- The patient denies sexual activity, but has clearly been sexually active in the past (gravida 2, para 0).
- I need to carry out urinalysis to rule out pregnancy as a cause.
- Pregnancy test (bHCG) positive.
- Pain in early pregnancy carries risk of ectopic presentation.
- I cannot manage this presentation in this setting.
- This patient needs to go to hospital urgently.

Ethical Considerations

This patient is potentially vulnerable and should be subject to a safeguarding referral.

Professional Issues

This case highlights the importance of professional insight and a willingness to determine one's own limitations, but this does not need to diminish good decision making. Having weaknesses in certain areas (such as, in this case, learning disabilities) drives learning and reflection, and does not infer a lack of wider competency. Paramedics are arguably best described against the literature as 'generalists/extended generalists' (Benner, 1984), and may not be exposed to patients such as this on a regular basis.

The Best Outcome Using Good Decision-making Processes

The patient attended the emergency department at the local hospital and underwent further blood and urine tests to confirm pregnancy. An ultrasound scan showed the pregnancy was ectopic and at risk of rupture. The patient went to the operating room later that day and went on to make a full recovery. She went home a few days later and met with her support worker and social worker to ensure that the relationship she is in is appropriate and to offer specific support relating to her sexual health.

Decision-making Assessment and Key Learning Points

Relying on logical decision making can help overcome any gaps by applying the same processes consistently and challenging information critically rather than simply accepting what you hear. Abdominal pain in females of child-bearing age carries the same physical health risks for any patient suffering with it, regardless of any other circumstance, and introducing a learning disability provides an example of how the principles of good decision making can overcome additional complexities by processing the data and turning the 'what' into 'why'. Imagine if the paramedic had accepted the patient's denial of sexual activity as a 'what' and therefore treated it as a fact – this would have been a fork in the road early on in the encounter, which would inform all other decisions, and is therefore critical. Think back to the bagatelle board example in Chapter 5, and consider the focus of possible differential diagnoses in the absence of pregnancy-related issues. It's vital to ask yourself 'why' the patient gave the answer she gave, and to challenge yourself to ensure that you understood it in the way the patient intended. Patients may use euphemisms or other colloquialisms to describe things to avoid embarrassment, or because it was a term used in childhood. We should ensure that we learn to receive information rather than expect patients to present it in our preferred way.

There are references in this book that encourage a level of healthy scepticism when analysing data, and this must be balanced against ensuring that we build and maintain trust between us and our patient, but sometimes patients may not be able or willing to give the answer we expect for a variety of reasons.

Case Study 6: 23-year-old Female Car Crash

Background

You are working in the out of hospital environment and receive a 911 call for a car that has left the road, rolled over and landed in the water on its wheels. You arrive to the address and are met by bystanders that are glad you have arrived . You made it to scene fairly quickly after the call was made. The car struck a tree before landing in the sea water with high tide due in 2 hours. The car is submerged to the level of the windows with what appears to have minimal intrusion to the driving compartment. The driver extricated their passenger and both driver and passenger were found by bystanders lying on the side of the road.

> HPC: The patient was driving with their partner and was not able to navigate the sharp turn at their rate of speed.

PMHx: Depression.

DH: Unknown.

Allergies: NKDA.

SH: Independent young female.

SE: Unknown LOC, pain in midline cervical spine upon palpation, rapid body survey is unremarkable, tearful and anxious. No other obvious bony injury felt head to toe, chest, abdomen and long bones are all intact. Skin is wet and cold.

O/E: Observations within normal parameters, no obvious neurology, no paraesthesia or lack of tone or power, active shivering.

Imp: Neck pain.

Plan: Consider spinal motion restriction when recent experiences have demonstrated no need for restriction based on transporting paramedics.

Potential Outcome for This Patient with Poor Decision Making

Intuitive Responses

The patient isn't keen at all transport to hospital, she is quite eager to see her mom and get on with her evening and is sorry for making a fuss. The paramedics often do not place a c-collar and immobilize the spine after the patient's ambulate. *Common things are common.* I appreciate there is chance for serious injury here, but in spite of being emotional the patient seems sensible enough for me to allow her to walk to the stretcher for transport and apply a c-collar then.

Biases and Fallacies

Review the section on 'Human Fallibility and Biased Thinking' in Chapter 3 to find the biases used in the example.

- **Neglect of probability** – The chance of serious injury is small but still needs to be considered.
- **Averages bias** – how often are we performing procedures that may or may not be warranted.
- **Overconfidence bias** – this decision has been made successfully before based on previous experience and this is the same.

Actual Outcome for This Patient with Poor Decision Making

The patient presents to their GP 2 weeks later with increasing neck pain. The GP sends her for imaging, which shows a fractured cervical spine. The facture is stable, but if the patient had been walked to the ambulance, this could have resulted in a more serious outcome.

Professional Insights

- Of the screening tools I have available, is this a safe decision?
- What are the tools or diagnostics that I do not have access to in this environment to develop the appropriate care plan?
- What are the risks of not treating with spinal motion restriction?
- What other potential risks or diagnoses am I missing?

Human Factors

- Is the decision maker well rested enough to make a good decision?
- The patient is keen to get on with the rest of her day. Spinal motion restriction will require a bit more work, do I really want to do that?
- 'Blissful ignorance' – Lack of education and appreciation for likely injury. Likely cofounded by years of practice with no feedback loop for similar presentations.

Deductive Reasoning

The client has had a mechanism that is highly suspicious of a cervical spine fracture due to a motor vehicle collision, at rate of speed resulting in at least one roll, and midline c-spine tenderness. Her high anxiety makes it challenging to establish if there are any distractions to her injuries.The fact she is complaining of neck pain is a red flag. Although she has no neurology and this is likely to be a stable fracture, it still requires spinal motion restriction until diagnostic imaging confirms presence and/or degree of injury.

Decision-making Assessment and Key Learning Points

The decision making here is complex. Has the client sustained a bony injury to the cervical spine or is this a musculature injury? Is the patient distracted by their environment and temperature after being in the water? Is she worried and anxious about her partner that was also in the vehicle? There is a growing body of knowledge that supports moving away from spinal motion restriction and the use of rigid collars. There are also a few tools that can be chosen by paramedics to aid in this decision making. It can be challenging to manage the risks associated with this sort of decision. From an **average bias** perspective, more often than not, it appears as though spinal motion restriction is not required, perhaps this presentation is no different? From a paramedic experiential perspective or intuition, perhaps the mechanism wasn't that bad? We have seen this before, performed spinal motion restriction when it wasn't required and therefore this time is no different. There are red flags in this patient encounter. Is the patient distracted with an emotional state of being or the cold environment. Is the patient mildly hypothermic? Is it safe and have you mitigated the risk appropriately by not providing spinal motion restriction? There are limitations to paramedic practice especially when context and environment are considered. Given your examination and findings of pinpoint cervical spine tenderness, an altered or distracted state of being and a mechanism of injury, many risks will need to be managed with diagnostics that are not available in this context of practice.

Case Study 7: 40-year-old Male with GI Bleed

Background

You are working in the ED as the department critical care paramedic and are asked to perform a procedural sedation for a GI scope secondary to a GI bleed.

- HPC: David has a 4-month history of left-sided abdominal (LUQ) pain radiating to the back with vomiting, seen in ED previously last month, where the symptoms were thought to be due to constipation (bloods were unremarkable). Symptoms are persisting episodically, despite increasing fibre intake, which occasionally helps. The patient often feels bloated and struggles to pass bowel movements. More recently, David is now experiencing more severe pain that seems to be radiating down his abdomen, and yesterday has lost his appetite as eating exacerbates the pain. He is becoming increasingly concerned that something sinister is happening. He is beginning to lose sleep.
- PMH: None.
- Allergies: NKDA.
- DH: None, has been taking OTC Fybogel and PRN acetaminophen. Occasionally drinks, is a non-smoker.
- SH: Lives with family, works a stressful job and might be facing redundancy.
- SE: Otherwise well. Feels constipated, symptoms thought to resolve after passing bowels. No weight loss. Stool is reported as normal.
- OE: HR 98 and regular; BP 100/78 mmHg; RR 20; SpO_2 98%; Temp 36.5°C. Looks unwell. Abdomen visually normal, slightly overweight. ASA 3 (severe dysfunctional disease and some functional limitaitons). You have reviewed routine blood work and note a low haemoglobin with no transfusions noted.
- IMP: High risk patient for procedural sedation, defer or request the addition of anesthesia.
- Plan: Discussion of concerns with charge physician results in a request to move forward with the sedation.

Potential Outcome for This Patient with Poor Decision Making

Intuitive Responses

Given both the number of sedations you have completed and that are performed in the emergency department and their associated success rate, the incident of adverse events is unlikely. I am probably just nervous about performing GI sedations given the required positioning of the patient and limited access to the airway with the scope being introduced PO. The charge physician would know best, so we should proceed *Try and reflect on what you thought intuitively when reading this case.*

Bias and Human Factors

There is an action bias, overconfidence bias and authority bias present within this case – There was a need for the team to identify the source of the bleeding with this patient and perhaps a need to do something about it, to find the source. The cornerstone of the critical care paramedic ED practice has been their ability to safely assess patients that can undergo procedural sedation and analgesia – historically with very few adverse events; surely this sedation would result in a positive outcome. Finally, although the department paramedic objectively identified risks to performing the procedural sedation in the ED, the charge physician with higher authority within the department, excused the identified risks.

Outcome with Poor Decision Making

The patient was prepared for the procedural sedation; the sedation was initiated and the GI team proceeded with their scope. Early in the procedure despite adequate preoxygenation, and preloading of volume with crystalloid and the careful administration of sedation, the patient developed hypotension and a drop in oxygen saturation. The scope was discontinued and the patient was successfully resuscitated by the paramedic. The scope was delayed until the patient was further resuscitated with blood transfusion.

Two hours post transfusion and follow up CBC result in a positive trending haemoglobin; the procedural sedation and GI scope was completed.

Outcome with Good Decision Making

A huddle that included the charge physician, GI team lead and paramedic allowed for a conversation where factors that were identified as high risk to having a procedural sedation performed were discussed. This discussion supported a shared mental model on the current state of the patient and suggested intervention.

The collaborative team agreed that an attempt to resuscitate the patient with blood prior to sedation would be in the best interest of the patient. The patient received two untis of blood and raised their MAP enough to safely prepare the patient for the sedation. The sedation moved forward without adverse event and the patient received clips at various bedding sites upon their GI scope.

Information Processing (Critical Analysis of Data and Information)

- As a proceduralist, you recognize risks based on exam, pharmacodynamics and hemodynamics, are these being shared with the charge physician?

- Is there a safer option with similar outcomes? Have they been discussed or shared with the team?
- Are there human factors of other teammates that may be factoring into the decision? Hunger/anger/late/lonely/tired?
- Flank pain indicates a renal cause and ought to be investigated in further depth.

Professional Insights

- Although you are confident that you can complete the procedural sedation, this appears to be a high risk, and could benefit from an additional team member, a better environment (OR) and/or defer the procedure for further resuscitation prior to the sedation being completed.
- Given the ASA score and the assessment, is this the appropriate place for this patient to be receiving a procedural sedation for the GI scope?
- Can I manage this sedation, or should anesthesia perform this procedure?
- Have I objectively communicated the risks identified? Do I need to escalate the level of concern in my communication approach?

Hypotheses/Differential Diagnoses (With Positive Features –!)

- Anemia
- Hypovolemia
- Hypovolemic shock

Deductive Reasoning

- David has a reduced oxygen carrying capacity that requires consideration.
- Procedural sedation carries a risk of reducing MAP.
- Does this need to be acted on immediately?
- There are other options to consider given the risks of proceeding immediately.

Ethical Considerations

- **Non-maleficence** – Does David require a GI scope? Is the risk of David receiving the GI scope in the ED now worth it versus delaying the scope post resuscitation or moving to the OR?
- **Justice** – Am I about to perform a procedure to David unnecessarily? Am I the best clinician to be performing this procedure?

Professional Issues

- Difficult conversation with charge physician – create an environment where your concerns are heard and appreciated.
- Evaluate risks and benefits, is this the safest place for this procedure to occur? If not, advocate for patient on behalf of the risk benefits.

The Best Outcome Using Good Decision-making Processes

Based on your physical examination of David and your understanding of the risks associated with a procedural sedation for a GI scope in an under resuscitated patient, a team huddle was performed and there was a shared decision to administer an additional unit of packed cells. The team agreed that this should manage the risks appropriately and the ED would be appropriate for the GI scope as opposed to needed to book for an OR.

The procedural sedation was performed by the emergency department paramedic allowing the GI scope team to place three clips to manage Davids upper GI bleed. When David's hemodynamics improved, Davis was transferred to a bed within the hospital for follow up care and monitoring.

Decision Making: Assessment and Key Learning Points

David's case highlights the importance of recognizing an authority bias and utilizing a shared decision approach to safely provide care and work to overcome barriers to critical thinking that may emerge.

- In this particular instance, a reliance on intuition alone does not support critical thinking and one's ability to discuss safe options to provide the care David requires.
- Additionally, not being open to other safe options (absolutism) to providing care is not beneficial to David. Given David's ASA score, an argument may have been made to perform the sedation in the OR. Collectively, a safe alternative was achieved allowing for the procedural sedation to be completed in the ED.
- Authority bias can be challenging to navigate. There are various approaches that can be used to create space for shared decision making and to allow teams to function in a dynamic that allows for unput from anyone on the team regardless of 'rank'.
- The Garden Gate Test has some applicability in David's case. If you are leaving the room and are already considering consequences of things that may go wrong – you have made the wrong decision. Although confidence complicates this somewhat, there is value in ensuring that you have made a robust decision by considering the Garden Gate Test

Perhaps on a closing note, considering the context of others when communicating about decisions may contribute to making a paramedic a better communicator, particularly in difficult situations when making difficult decisions. As identified in Chapter 4, the way you communicate with your body language, the terminology you choose, the setting you choose to communicate within and your willingness to listen (not hear) your teammates impacts communication and performance. Science has demonstrated to healthcare, including paramedicine, that improved team performance improves patient care.

Appendix

Regulatory Practice Standards Published by the Canadian Organization of Paramedic Regulators

1. Scope of Practice
2. Competence
3. Cultural Safety and Humility
4. Privacy and Confidentiality
5. Professional Boundaries
6. Duty to Report
7. Patient Assessment, Diagnosis, and Interventions
8. Communications
9. Collaboration and Professional Relationships
10. Documentation and Record Keeping

Glossary

Absolutism Application of an idea or principle to the exclusion of other considerations.

Acuity Acuteness or sharpness. In healthcare it usually refers to the severity of a patient's condition (for example, 'polytrauma patients are high acuity').

Acumen Astuteness. Often used in reference to developing an ability or knowledge. In this book, we refer to building decision-making acumen.

Aetiology The cause, or nature of cause, of a disease. For example, the link between obesity and diabetes.

Affect heuristics Intuitive responses able to be completed competently but influenced by emotion, such as when someone reacts to a car backfiring by running away prior to realizing it isn't gunfire. The turning and running is the heuristic ability and the emotion (fear) provides the affect.

Agency The capacity to act. Often used interchangeably with autonomy and linked closely with biomedical ethics.

Allied health professionals The group of healthcare professionals led by the Chief Allied Health Professions Office within NHS England. Distinct from medicine and nursing.

Anterior ST segment elevation A very specific interpretation on an electrocardiogram of the anterior view (leads V3 and V4), which typically indicates a myocardial infarction but can also indicate other cardiovascular instability.

Anthropometrics Designing something with the end user's comfort in mind. For example, ensuring a worktop is at the correct height to prevent stooping.

Authority bias Being influenced by someone by dint of their rank or seniority, rather than being right or wrong.

Autonomy Able to be self-governing. Different from agency, but often used interchangeably. Autonomy is more the right to self-determination, whereas agency is the ability or capacity to act.

Availability bias A mental shortcut to connect ideas (heuristics) and decisions that are readily available so as to exclude alternatives (also known as the unknown).

Base-rate neglect Ignoring the baseline information upon which context is derived. For example, believing that all immigrants are criminals because 75% of crimes in an area were carried out by immigrants, regardless of the number of immigrants in the area or how many crimes were carried out by the same people. The baseline is the immigrant population, and the crime statistics should be considered in light of the baseline (base rate) rather than in isolation.

Beneficence An act that is undertaken for a patient's benefit. Beneficent acts may prevent harm or further harm, and/or can be used to improve the patient's situation.

bHCG test Beta Human Gonadotrophic Hormone blood or urine test. The bHCG hormone is produced only in pregnancy and its presence indicates the patient is pregnant. May return a false positive, but rarely a false negative unless tested too early in pregnancy.

Biomedical ethics Refers to the examination of the ethics of all biomedical research, medicine and healthcare.

Cognition Mental action or process of acquiring knowledge and understanding. Using your brain to provide an answer or solution; working something out; deducing.

Cognitive continuum The gradient between scientific enquiry and pure intuition relating to decision making.

Cognitive dissonance The discomfort felt when a person has two competing beliefs regarding a particular issue or concept, leading to contradiction and internal conflict – particularly when considering new evidence.

Cognitive tasks Tasks needing cognitive input (thoughts, considerations, judgements). Mental arithmetic, for example.

Collaborative decision making Working with patients, families, carers, colleagues, other agencies to develop the best outcome for patients based on informed choice. May be used more specifically in the context of patients as 'shared decision making' or with other professionals as 'shared professional decision making'.

Co-morbid/co-morbidity Diseases that a patient has or acquires on top of an existing disease. For instance, if a patient with heart failure then develops dementia, the dementia is the co-morbidity.

Confirmation bias Using information or evidence to support pre-existing beliefs or decisions – often selectively (i.e., a normal ECG in the patient with chest pain does not in isolation support the conclusion that the patient is not having a heart attack).

Conformism A conformist tends to follow the prevailing culture, beliefs or standards and may not question or challenge.

Conjunction bias Conjoining concepts in a convenient way – leaping to conclusions.

Contractualism In ethics, the school of thought that human beings hold invisible contracts (predominantly on a social level) with each other that affect our moral actions in some way. Elements include the responsibility to look after others as well as ourselves, or the basic access to health and education, while also balancing equality and liberty.

Defensibly Decisions that can be reasonably justified, even in unexpected outcomes.

Defensive practice Basing decisions that cannot be challenged as unsafe. Examples include over-investigation and unnecessary conveyance.

Demography Data on the composition of populations, including births, deaths, income, epidemiology.

Deontology/deontological ethics Duty or obligation. Judgements of actions based on normative rules. For instance, the reasonable assumption, as well as prevailing laws, that killing people is morally wrong.

Descriptive decision theory Explores decisions that ought to be made based on a prevalent disposition. In essence, some decisions can be predictable.

Diagnostic reasoning Often referred to as 'clinical decision making'. Links the specific ability to use the tools described in this book to make a diagnosis.

Duty of Care Refers to the obligations placed on people to act towards others in a reasonable way, in accordance with certain standards. These standards were initially derived from the works of Kant, in which all individuals deserve respect and dignity.

Encephalitis Swelling of the brain.

Encephalopathy Conditions that affect brain functioning, such as disease or injury.

Epidemiology The study of disease prevalence among populations, for example, coronary heart disease in different towns and cities in a country. May be linked to demography and levels of deprivation.

Epistemology The theory of knowledge and its acquisition.

Ergonomics Designing things to be efficient and comfortable.

Error In decision making, due to a mixture of bias, competence (skill or knowledge), and situational attitude.

Ethnocentrism The belief that one's own group or culture is superior to other groups.

Experiential A word that describes knowledge based on experience or observation. Often used to infer superiority of knowledge and skills. Experience should be consolidated and reflected upon.

False causality bias The incorrect assumption that sequential events are linked. In the decision-making context, an example is assuming that a 3-day history of coughing is the cause of the patient's chest pain, when in fact the patient is having a heart attack. This bias features heavily when considering purely intuitive decision making.

Gatekeeping The act of controlling access to something. In healthcare, this is typically access to specialist services. A clear example for ambulances is the decision to convey to a stroke unit.

Groupthink The situation where a group of people create a consensus that other members of the group may fail to challenge, even if the consensus is wrong. People tend to not speak out rather than risk being wrong, or being seen as an outsider or opposed to the view of the group.

HCPC The Health and Care Professions Council, the regulator for 14 health and social care professions in the UK. The HCPC is overseen by the PSA (Professional Standards Authority), which also oversees the General Medical Council (GMC) and the Nursing and Midwifery Council (NMC).

Hermeneutics The theory and methodology of text interpretation, especially the interpretation of biblical texts, wisdom literature and philosophical texts. Hermeneutics was initially applied to the interpretation, or exegesis, of scripture.

Hernia Where an organ protrudes through the wall of the cavity containing it. The most common hernias are inguinal, where a small length of intestine protrudes through the inguinal canal.

Heuristics Obtaining knowledge through experimentation (trial and error) leading to tacit understanding sufficient to solve most issues relating to the subject. Essentially pattern recognition.

Holistic Treatment of the 'whole person' rather than just the disease, and includes mental/psychological and social needs and considerations.

Human factors The influence environments and systems have on human beings, which can lead to errors or other issues.

Hypothesis An idea put forward for testing deductively. Differential diagnoses are hypotheses in the healthcare setting.

Hypothetico-deduction A process of scientific enquiry used to test hypotheses in order to reach the correct answer.

Ideation The formation of ideas. In healthcare, it may be used in context to mental health crises where a patient expresses 'suicidal ideation' – suggesting that they are forming ideas about possible ways to end their life.

Illusory superiority An overestimation of one's ability. There are lots of examples in healthcare, where this can lead to risk of harm to patients. An example in life in general may be experienced when you hear someone say, 'Hold my beer!'

Intuitionism A theory of ethics in which moral decisions are derived from what feels right on the face of things (*prima facie*). These feelings can then develop into a moral code of thinking (wisdom) for future situations.

Ischaemic bowel Loss of blood supply to the bowel, leading to loss of function and death of the section of bowel. May lead to peritonitis and can be fatal.

Just culture The promotion of fairness, openness and learning, encouraging individuals to speak up when things go wrong rather than fearing blame.

Justice In relation to biomedical ethics, justice is defined as the patient receiving what is minimally reasonable or should be expected in terms of care, treatment and level of service (given what is available). It can also be considered as what is owed to the patient.

Known knowns That which you are confident that you know to the point where you can demonstrate the knowledge to yourself or others.

Known unknowns Subjects that you know you do not have sufficient knowledge of. Clinicians who can express their known unknowns are demonstrating good levels of insight into their own practice and are less prone to illusory superiority.

Latent error Contributory factors, or smaller cumulative errors, which can lead to larger-scale issues, but which are often overlooked.

Learning culture/no blame culture Organizations that seek to learn from untoward incidents and errors are said to have a 'no blame' and/or 'learning culture'. Assigning blame rarely addresses the true root cause of an error or incident, and sharing learning is vital to ensure incidents are not repeated. This can only happen where clinicians feel sufficiently safe to report errors and incidents.

Logical intuition Considered essentially as common sense, which is less susceptible to bias.

Loss aversion The preference to avoid losing rather than trying to achieve gain. It is preferable not to lose a £10 note than to find a £10 pound note.

Mental capacity An individual's ability to make their own choices and decisions.

Morbidity The condition of being diseased. Having a disease or injury, or a condition considered pathological (i.e., morbid obesity – the obesity is such that it is affecting the patient's normal function as though they were sick or injured).

Multi-morbidity The presence of two or more major diseases at the same time. Different from co-morbidity in that there is more than one primary condition being treated actively.

Murphy's sign A physical assessment technique used to identify pain in the gall bladder.

Myocardial infarction Blockage of a coronary artery impairing blood flow to the heart muscle, leading to ischaemia and loss of function. Can lead to cardiac arrest and death.

Nonmaleficence 'Do no harm'. Ensuring that the treatment being given will not cause greater discomfort or risk to the patient without due consideration of the benefits.

Normative decision theory That decisions should be optimal based on competing alternatives. Essentially why and how decisions are made.

Obturator test A physical assessment technique that elicits irritation of the *obturator internus* muscle and helps with the diagnosis of appendicitis.

Over-testing More testing than necessary to diagnose patients with signs or symptoms. An example is blood capillary glucose testing in conscious patients without a history of diabetes, seizure or transient loss of consciousness.

Polypharmacy The prescribing of four or more medicines to patients aged over 65. Polypharmacy is associated with other risks to the patient, such as increased risk of falling.

Positivism Only recognizing that which can be proven scientifically, and rejecting concepts such as theism and meta-physics.

Post-positivist Amends positivism such that human knowledge is a combination of human perspectives as well as experimental evidence.

Principlism The foremost normative decision theory in bioethics. More commonly known as the combination of the 'four principles' of beneficence, non-maleficence, justice and autonomy in determining a morally sound decision.

Psoas sign A physical assessment technique that elicits irritation in the iliopsoas group of hip flexor muscles in the abdomen. It helps identify the location of the appendix relative to the caecum.

Quasi-rationality 'Quasi' means something resembling another concept. The term 'rationality' simply means that something was done for, or with, reason.

Reasonable alternatives The consideration of alternative plausible actions before the final decision is made. In paramedic practice, common reasonable alternatives include GP or senior referral, non-conveyance with self-care (depending on the patient presentation) and conveyance to hospital.

Right iliac fossa A depression in the right iliac region of the abdomen where pain or tenderness may be elicited in the presence of appendicitis commonly.

ROSC Return of spontaneous circulation. Successfully restarting a patient's heart who has been in cardiac arrest sufficient for the patient's circulation to support itself.

Rote learning Learning that is achieved through habitual or repetitive study, and occasionally without the underpinning understanding. For example, learning times tables at school without learning why or how to make calculation easier.

Rovsing's test A physical assessment technique used to assist in the diagnosis of appendicitis. It involves palpating the left lower quadrant in order to elicit pain in the right lower quadrant.

Shared decision making Decision making that usually takes place between patient and clinician during care planning or other decision making about treatment. It can also refer to the collaborative decision making between clinicians used to assist clinicians working in isolation.

Sociocentricity Focus on one's own social group or culture. Parochialism.

Socratic paradox This paradox provides the origin of the four statements relating to knowledge: I know what I know; I know what I don't know; I don't know what I know; I don't know what I don't know.

Suturing Closure of a wound using sutures (stitches).

System-1 thinking Fast, intuitive thinking, often heuristical (patterns), unconscious or based on a feeling.

System-2 thinking Slow, deliberate thinking.

Tacit knowledge The ability to apply prior heuristics or actions to differing situations that are similar in presentation. The process of cardiopulmonary resuscitation from an experienced paramedic is an example of this.

Task-cycle time The time taken to complete one patient encounter and be subsequently available for the next. It can also be known more colloquially as job-cycle.

Thought experiments The creation of an imaginative scenario in order to test theories in the mind.

Utilitarianism In its simplest form is the greatest happiness for the greatest number of people. It is a consequentialist theory in which benefit is measured on the outcome of an action.

Veil of ignorance Assuming you have no knowledge of position in society (rich or poor), how would you like society to be shaped? What limited resources should be available to whom? This is the veil of ignorance, which serves as a thought experiment on the distribution of resources.

Virtue ethics Concerns the ability of the individual to make good moral decisions based on virtuous characteristics (honesty, compassion and courage, for instance), rather than focusing on duty or consequence of actions.

YLD Years Lived with Disability. Years Lived with Disability is a metric which combines the severity of a disease's symptoms (excluding death itself) with its prevalence, to measure its impact on quality of life.

Bibliography

Abwalaba, R.A. and Onyango, P.O. (2019). Competence of paramedics in the management of emergency conditions in Kisumu County, Kenya. *International Journal of Education and Research*, 7(7): 149–158.

Adler, R., Rosenfeld, L. and Proctor, R. (2001). *Interplay: The Process of Interpersonal Communicating*, 8th edn. Fort Worth, TX: Harcourt. Available: https://relivingmbadays.wordpress.com/2013/04/04/listening-skills-2/ (accessed 09 January 2024).

Agan, R.D. (1987). Intuitive knowing as a dimension of nursing. *Advances in Nursing Science*, 10(1): 63–70.

Air Accidents Investigation Branch (AAIB) (2021). Air Accidents Investigation Branch. Available: https://www.gov.uk/government/organisations/air-accidents-investigation-branch (accessed 09 January 2024).

Allied Health Professions Federation (AHPF) (2021). Member Organisations. Available: http://www.ahpf.org.uk/member_organisations.htm (accessed 09 January 2024).

American Academy of Orthopaedic Surgeons (AAOS) (2022). *Nancy Caroline's Emergency Care in the Streets*, 9th edn. Burlington, MA: Jones & Bartlett Learning.

Ancona, D. (2012). Sensemaking: Framing and Acting in the Unknown. In S. Snook, N. Nohria & R. Khur (Eds), *The Handbook for Teaching Leadership: Knowing, Doing, and Being*. Los Angeles: Sage, pp. 3–19.

Anderson, N.E., Slark, J. and Gott, M. (2021). Prehospital Resuscitation Decision Making: A model of ambulance personnel experiences, preparation and support. *Emergency Medicine Australasia*, *33*(4), pp. 697–702.

Ariely, D. (2023). *Misbelief*. New York: Harper Collins.

Ashforth, B.E., Harrison, S.H. and Corley, K.G. (2008). Identification in organizations: An examination of four fundamental questions. *Journal of Management*, 34: 325–374. Available: http://leeds-faculty.colorado.edu/dahe7472/Journal%20of%20Management-2008-Ashforth-325-74.pdf (accessed 09 January 2024).

Aviation Safety Network. (n.d.). Tenerife Air Accident Resources. [Online]. Aviation Safety Network. Available at: https://aviation-safety.net/database/record.php?id=19770327-1 [accessed 18 February 2024].

Babbage, C. (1864). *Passages from the Life of a Philosopher*. London: Longman and Co.

Baines Simmons Ltd (2019). FAIR3® A Behaviour-based System for Supporting and Sustaining a Just Culture. Available: https://www.bainessimmons.com/aviation-consulting-services/smarrt-tools/fair-system/ (accessed 09 January 2024).

Banks, S. and Gallagher, A. (2008). *Ethics in Professional Life: Virtues for Health and Social Care*. Basingstoke: Palgrave Macmillan.

Barber, B., (1963). Some problems in the sociology of the professions. *Daedalus*, pp. 669–688.

Baron, J. (2006). *Against Bioethics*. Cambridge, MA: MIT Press, p. xi.

Bartlett, K.R., (2001). The relationship between training and organizational commitment: A study in the health care field. *Human resource development quarterly*, 12(4), pp. 335–352.

Bastick, T. (1982). *How We Think and Act*. New York: John Wiley.

Beauchamp, T.L. and Childress, J.F. (2019) *Principles of biomedical ethics*, 8th edn. New York: Oxford University Press.

Becker, T.K., Martin-Gill, C., Callaway, C.W., Guyette, F.X. and Schott, C. (2017). Feasibility of paramedic performed prehospital lung ultrasound in medical patients with respiratory distress. *Prehospital Emergency Care*, 22(2): 175–179.

Benner, P. (1984). *From Novice to Expert*. Menlo Park, CA: Addison-Wesley.

Benner, P. and Tanner, C. (1987). Clinical judgement: How expert nurses use intuition. *American Journal of Nursing*, 87(1): 23–34.

Blaber, A. (2008). *Foundations for Paramedic Practice: A Theoretical Perspective*. London: McGraw Hill.

Blackmore, T. (Ed.). (2022). *Palliative and end of Life Care for paramedics*. Bridgwater: Class Professional Publishing

Bonner, A. (2003). Recognition of expertise: An important concept in the acquisition of nephrology nursing expertise. *Nursing and Health Sciences*, 5(2): 123–131.

Bordage, G. (1999). Why did I miss the diagnosis? Some cognitive explanations and educational implications. *Academic Medicine*, 74(10): S138–142.

Bowles, R., van Beek, C., Anderson, G. (2017). Four dimensions of paramedic practice in Canada: Defining and describing the profession. *Australasian Journal of Paramedicine*, 14(3).

Braithwaite, S. (2014). Ethics in paramedic practice: A qualitative case study of paramedic perceptions of ethical decision-making in practice. Doctoral Thesis, North Carolina State University.

Brandolini, A. (2013). Brandolini's law. Available: https://twitter.com/ziobrando/status/289635060758507521 (accessed 09 January 2024).

Bravo, P., Edwards, A., Barr, P.J., Scholl, I., Elwyn, G. and McAllister, M. (2015). Conceptualising patient empowerment: a mixed methods study. *BMC health services research*, *15*(1), pp. 1–14.

British Geriatrics Society (BGS) (2017). Deconditioning Awareness. Available: https://www.bgs.org.uk/resources/deconditioning-awareness (accessed 09 January 2024).

Broadwell, M.M. (1969). Teaching for learning (XVI). The Gospel Guardian. Available: https://wordsfitlyspoken.org/gospel_guardian/v20/v20n41p1-3a.html (accessed 09 January 2024).

Broockman, D. and Kalla, J. (2016). Durably reducing transphobia: A field experiment on door-to-door canvassing. *Science*, 352(6282): 220–224. Available: https://science.sciencemag.org/content/352/6282/220 (accessed 09 January 2024).

Brush, J. (2015). *The Science of the Art of Medicine*. Virginia: Dementi Milestone Publishing.

Cambridge Dictionary (2021). Available at: http://dictionary.cambridge.org/dictionary/english (accessed 09 January 2024).

Cameron, C. and Batt, A.M. (2024). *Career Framework for Paramedics* (1st edition). Ottawa: Paramedic Association of Canada. Available at: https:// doi.org/10.17605/osf.io/wdh9m (accessed 27 February 2026).

Canadian Encyclopedia. (2026). Elder Albert Marshall. Available: https://www.thecanadianencyclopedia.ca/en/article/albert-marshall (accessed 29 April 2026)

Care Quality Commission. (2014). Regulation 18: Staffing. [Online]. Care Quality Commission. Last Updated: August 2023. Available at: https://www.cqc.org.uk/guidance-providers/regulations/regulation-18-staffing [accessed 18 February 2024].

Carnevali, D.L., Mitchell, P.H., Woods, N.F. and Tanner, C.A. (1984). *Diagnostic Reasoning in Nursing*. Philadelphia, PA: Lippincott.

Carper, B. (1978). Fundamental ways of knowing in nursing. *Advances in Nursing Science*, 1(1): 13–23.

Carter of Coles, Lord and NHS Ambulance Trusts (2018). Operational Productivity and Performance in English NHS Ambulance Trusts: Unwarranted Variations. Available: https://www.england.nhs.uk/wp-content/uploads/2019/09/Operational_productivity_and_performance_NHS_Ambulance_Trusts_final.pdf (accessed 09 January 2024).

Charlin, B., Tardif, J. and Boshuizen, H.P.A. (2000). Scripts and medical diagnostic knowledge: Theory and applications for clinical reasoning instruction and research. *Academic Medicine*, 75(2): 182–190.

Chartered Institute of Ergonomics and Human Factors. (2020). *White Paper: Learning from Adverse Events*. Warwickshire, UK: Chartered Institute of Ergonomics and Human Factors.

Christensen, M. and Hewitt-Taylor, J. (2006). From expert to tasks, expert nursing practice redefined? *Issues in Clinical Nursing*, 15(12): 1531–1539.

Cianfrani, K.L. (1984). The influence of amounts and relevance of data on identifying health problems. In: Kim, M.J., McFarland, G.K. and McLane, A.M. (eds). *Classifications of Nursing Diagnoses: Proceedings of the Fifth National Conference*. St Louis, MO: Mosby.

Cioffi, J. (1997). Heuristics, servants to intuition, in clinical decision making. *Journal of Advanced Nursing*, 26: 203–208.

Cioffi, J. (2002). What are clinical judgements? In: Thompson, C. and Dowding, D. (eds). *Clinical Decision Making and Judgement in Nursing*. Edinburgh: Churchill Livingstone.

Civility Saves Lives (n.d.) Our Message. Available from: https://www.civilitysaveslives.com/our-message (accessed 09 January 2024).

Clack, G. (2009). Decision making in nursing practice: A case review. *Paediatric Nursing*, 21(5): 24–27.

Clinical Human Factors Group (CHFG) (2015). Human Factors in Healthcare: Common Terms. Available: https://chfg.org/human-factors-in-healthcare-common-terms/ (accessed 09 January 2024).

College of Paramedics. (2024). The Paramedic Curriculum, 6th edn. Bridgwater: College of Paramedics. Available from: https://collegeofparamedics.co.uk/COP/ProfessionalDevelopment/Developing%20a%20New%20Paramedic%20Curriculum.aspx [Accessed 29 May 2024].

Communication Theory (n.d.). Shannon and Weaver Model of Communication. Available from: https://www.communicationtheory.org/shannon-and-weaver-model-of-communication/ (accessed 22 January 2024).

COPR (2025a). Canadian Organization of Paramedic Regulators. Available from: https://copr.ca/regulation-of-paramedics-canada/ (accessed 27 February 2026).

COPR (2025b). Pan-Canadian Essential Regulatory Requirements. Canadian Organization of Paramedic Regulators. Available from: https://copr.ca/regulation-of-paramedics-canada/ (accessed 27 February 2026).

Creton, D., Halter, M. and LaTrobe, C., (2020). A service evaluation of the experiences of specialist paramedics working in rotational environments using a retrospective cohort. Poster Presentation, *EMJ*, 37(10), p. 16.

Croskerry, P., (2009). A universal model of diagnostic reasoning. *Academic medicine*, 84(8), pp. 1022–1028.

CSA Group, (2024). National Standard of Canada: CSA Z1660:24. National Competency Framework for Paramedics.

Davey, P.J., Lees, A.B. and Godbold, R. (2016). Exploring New Zealand paramedic attitudes towards advance directives: An ethical analysis. *Australasian Journal of Paramedicine*, 13, 1–11.

Davis, J.K. (2007). Intuition and the junctures of judgment in decision procedures for clinical ethics. *Theoretical Medicine and Bioethics*, 28, 1–30.

DeJean, D., Giacomini, M., Welsford, M., Schwartz, L. and Decicca, P., (2016). Inappropriate ambulance use: a qualitative study of Paramedics' views. *Healthcare Policy*, 11(3), 67–79

De Neys, W. (2012). Bias and conflict a case for logical intuitions. *Perspectives on Psychological Science*, 7, 28–38.

De Neys, W. (2014). Conflict detection, dual processes, and logical intuitions: Some clarifications. *Thinking & Reasoning*, 20, 169–187.

Dees, R.H. (2019). *Primum non nocere mortuis*: Bioethics and the lives of the dead. *Journal of Medicine and Philosophy: A Forum for Bioethics and Philosophy of Medicine*, 44(6), 732–755.

Dekker, S. (2011). *Drift into Failure: From Hunting Broken Components to Understanding Complex Syst*. London: Routledge.

Dekker, S (2013). *Second Victim: Error, Guilt, Trauma, and Resilience*. London: Routledge.

Delizonna, L. (2017). High-performing teams need psychological safety: Here's how to create it. Six ways to build trust. *Harvard Business Review*. Available: https://hbr.org/2017/08/high-performing-teams-need-psychological-safety-heres-how-to-create-it (accessed 09 January 2024).

Department for Communities and Local Goverment. (2015). *The English Indices of Deprivation*. [Online]. UK Government. Available at: https://assets.publishing.service.gov.uk/media/5a7f42a940f0b6230268e6b3/English_Indices_of_Deprivati [accessed 02 March 2024].

Department for Transport (2014). Annual Road Fatalities. Available: www.gov.uk/government/publications/annual-road-fatalities (accessed 09 January 2024).

Department of Health (DH) (2005; 2011). *Taking Healthcare to the Patient: Transforming NHS Ambulance Services*. London: Department of Health.

Department of Health (DH) (2012). Long Term Conditions Compendium of Information, 3rd edn. Available: https://www.gov.uk/government/publications/long-term-conditions-compendium-of-information-third-edition (accessed 09 January 2024).

Department of Health (DH) (2015). 2010 to 2015 Government Policy: Long Term Health Conditions. Available: www.gov.uk/government/publications/2010-to-2015-government-policy-long-term-health-conditions/2010-to-2015-government-policy-long-term-health-conditions (accessed 09 January 2024).

Diekema, D.S. (2019). Decision making on behalf of children: Understanding the role of the harm principle. *Journal of Clinical Ethics*, 30(3): 207–212.

Dingley, C., Daugherty, K., Derieg, M.K. et al. (2008). Improving patient safety through provider communication strategy enhancements. In: Henriksen, K., Battles, J.B., Keyes, M.A. et al. (eds). *Advances in Patient Safety: New Directions and Alternative Approaches (Vol. 3: Performance and Tools)*. Rockville, MD: Agency for Healthcare Research and Quality (US). Available: https://www.ncbi.nlm.nih.gov/books/NBK43663/ (accessed 09 January 2024).

Dobelli, R. (2014). *The Art of Thinking Clearly*. London: Spectre.

Donabedian, A. (2005). Evaluating the Quality of Medical Care. *Millbank Quarterly*, 83(4): 691–729. Available: https://doi.org/10.1111%2Fj.1468-0009.2005.00397.x (accessed 09 January 2024).

Dowding, D., Spilsbury, K., Thompson, C., Brownlow, R. and Pattenden, J. (2009). The decision making of heart failure specialist nurses in clinical practice. *Journal of Clinical Nursing*, 18: 1313–1324.

Dowie, J. and Elstein, A. (1988). *Professional Judgement: A Reader in Clinical Decision Making*. Cambridge: Cambridge University Press.

Dreyfus, H.L. and Dreyfus, S. (1980). A five-stage model of the mental activities involved in direct skill acquisition. Unpublished Study, University of California, Berkeley, San Francisco, CA.

Dunning, D. and Kruger, J. (1999). Unskilled and unaware of it: How difficulties in recognizing one's own incompetence lead to inflated self-assessments. *Journal of Personality and Social Psychology*, 77(6): 1121–1134.

Easen, P. and Wilcockson, J. (1996). Intuition and rational decision-making in professional thinking: A false dichotomy. *Journal of Advanced Nursing*, 24: 667–673.

Eaton, G. (2024). *Law and Ethics for Paramedics: An Essential Guide*. 3rd edn. Bridgwater: Class Professional Publishing.

Ebben, R., van Vliet, R., Breedveld, L., Douwes, I., Hereijgers, J., van de Pas, H. and Vloet, L.C., (2020). Implementation of A Nurse Practitioner in Emergency Ambulance Care in The Netherlands: A Study Protocol for The IMPACT-Study.

Edwards, T.R., (2017). A prospective observational study to investigate the effect of prehospital airway management strategies on mortality and morbidity of patients who experience return of spontaneous circulation post cardiac arrest and are transferred directly to regional Heart Attack Centres by the Ambulance Service. Doctoral Thesis: University of Hertfordshire.

Einstein, A. (1933). On the method of theoretical physics. Lecture delivered at Oxford, 10 June 1933. Available: https://www.jstor.org/stable/184387 (accessed 09 January 2024).

Elliott, E., (2019). Normative decision theory. *Analysis*, *79*(4), pp. 755–772.

Elstein, A.S. and Schwarz, A. (2002). Clinical problem solving and diagnostic decision making: Selective review of the cognitive literature. *British Medical Journal*, 423(7339): 729–732.

Elstein, A.S., Shulman, L.S. and Sprafka, S.A. (1978). *Medical Problem Solving: An Analysis of Clinical Reasoning*. Cambridge, MA: Harvard University Press.

English, I. (1993). Intuition as a function of the expert nurse: A critique of Benner's Novice to Expert model. *Journal of Advanced Nursing*, 18: 387–393.

Equality Act (2010), Human Rights Act and the Public Sector Equality Duty.

Eraut, M. (1994). *Developing Professional Knowledge and Competence*. London: The Falmer Press.

F1 Stats. (2023). *Max Verstappen*. Available: https://www.statsf1.com/en/max-verstappen.aspx (accessed 09 January 2024).

FitzGerald, C., Martin, A., Berner, D. and Hurst, S. (2019). Interventions designed to reduce implicit prejudices and implicit stereotypes in real world contexts: A systematic review. *BMC Psychology*, 7(29). Available: https://bmcpsychology.biomedcentral.com/articles/10.1186/s40359-019-0299-7 (accessed 09 January 2024).

Freidson, E. (2001). *Professionalism: The Third Logic.* Chicago: University Chicago Press.

Gage, C.H., Geduld, H. and Stassen, W. (2020). South African paramedic perspectives on prehospital palliative care. *BMC Palliative Care*, 19(1): 1–11.

Gallagher, A., Vyvyan, E., Juniper, J., Snook, V., Horsfield, C., Collen, A. and Rutland, S. (2016). Consensus towards understanding and sustaining professionalism in paramedic practice. *British Paramedic Journal*, 1(2): 1–8.

Gambrill, E. (2012). *Critical Thinking in Clinical Practice*, 3rd edn. Hoboken, NJ: John Wiley.

Gardner, D. (2009). *Risk: The Science and Politics of Fear.* London: Virgin Books.

Geddes, J., Stewart, R., Baskett, T., (2017). T*he Evolution of Pre-Hospital Emergency Care Belfast and Beyond*. Bristol: Clinical Press Limited.

Gigerenzer, G. (2015). *Risk savvy: How to make good decisions*. New York: Penguin Random House.

Gilhooly, K.S. (1990). Cognitive psychology and medical diagnosis. *Applied Cognitive Psychology*, 4: 534–552.

Gillon, R. (2015). Defending the four principles approach as a good basis for good medical practice and therefore for good medical ethics. *Journal of Medical Ethics*, 41(1): 111–116.

Goode, W. J. (1960). Encroachment, Charlatanism and the Emerging Profession: Psychology, Sociology and Medicine. *American Sociological Review*, 25, 902–965.

Gopal, P. (2021). Implicit bias in healthcare: clinical practice, research and decision making. *Future Healthcare Journal*. 8(8), pp. 40–48. [Online]. Available at: https://doi.org/10.7861%2Ffhj.2020-0233 (accessed 27 April 2024).

Grant, J. and Marsden, P. (1987). The structure of memorized knowledge in students and clinicians: An explanation for diagnostic expertise. *Medical Education*, 21: 92.

Greenhalgh, T. and Hurwitz, B. (1998). *Narrative Based Medicine: Dialogue and Discourse in Clinical Practice*. London: BMJ Books.

Greenwood, B.N., Hardeman, R.R., Huang, L. and Sojourner, A. (2020). Physician–patient racial concordance and disparities in birthing mortality for newborns. *PNAS*, 117(35): 21194–21200. Available: https://www.pnas.org/content/117/35/21194 (accessed 09 January 2024).

Griffiths, B. (1978). Some comments on McDonald's paper. *Educational Studies in Mathematics*, 9: 87.

Griffin, B. and Smith, H. E., (2013). *Autobiography of Mark Twain*, Vol. 2, Berkley, CA: University of California Press.

Grunwald, I.Q., Phillips, D.J., Sexby, D., Wagner, V., Lesmeister, M., Bachhuber, M., Mathur, S., Guyler, P., Fisher, J., Perera, S. and Helwig, S.A., (2020). Mobile stroke unit in the UK healthcare system: avoidance of unnecessary accident and emergency admissions. *Cerebrovascular Diseases*, 49(4), pp. 388–395.

Hamers, J.P.H., Huijer Abu Saad, H. and Halfens, R.J.G. (1994). Diagnostic process and decision making in nursing: A literature review. *Journal of Professional Nursing*, 10(3): 154–163.

Hamm, R. (1988). Clinical intuition and clinical analysis: Expertise and the cognitive continuum. In: Dowie, J. and Eisten, A. (eds). *Professional Judgement: A Reader in Clinical Decision Making*. Cambridge: Cambridge University Press.

Hammond, K.R. (1981). *Principles of Organization in Intuitive and Analytical Cognition (Report 231*). Boulder, CO: Center for Research on Judgement and Policy, University of Colorado.

Hammond, K.R. (1996). *Human Judgement and Social Policy: Irreducible Uncertainty, Inevitable Error, Unavoidable Injustice*. New York: Oxford University Press.

Haney, C., Banks, W.C. and Zimbardo, P.G. (1973). A study of prisoners and guards in a simulated prison. *Naval Research Review*, 30: 4–17.

Harari, Y., Riemer, R., Jaffe, E., Wacht, O. and Bitan, Y. (2020). Paramedic equipment bags: How their position during out-of-hospital cardiopulmonary resuscitation (CPR) affects paramedic ergonomics and performance. *Applied Ergonomics*, 82: 102977.

Hawkridge, K., Ahmed, I. and Ahmed, Z., (2020). Evidence for the use of spinal collars in stabilising spinal injuries in the pre-hospital setting in trauma patients: a systematic review. *European Journal of Trauma and Emergency Surgery*, pp. 1–11.

Health and Care Professions Council (2014). *Standards of Proficiency: Paramedics*. HCPC: London. Available: https://www.hcpc-uk.org/globalassets/resources/standards/standards-of-proficiency---paramedics.pdf (accessed 09 January 2024).

Health and Care Professions Council (2016). Standards of Conduct, Performance and Ethics. Available: https://www.hcpc-uk.org/resources/standards/standards-of-conduct-performance-and-ethics/ (accessed 09 January 2024).

Health and Care Professions Council (2019). Indicative Sanctions Policy. Available: https://www.hcpc-uk.org/globalassets/consultations/2018/indicative-sanctions-policy/revised-indicative-sanctions-policy.pdf https://www.hcpc-uk.org/globalassets/resources/policy/sanctions-policy.pdf?v=637117389410000000 (accessed 09 January 2024).

Health and Care Professions Council (2020). Guidance on Confidentiality. Available: https://www.hcpc-uk.org/standards/meeting-our-standards/confidentiality/guidance-on-confidentiality/ (accessed 09 January 2024).

Health and Care Professions Council (2021). Record Keeping. Available: https://www.hcpc-uk.org/standards/meeting-our-standards/record-keeping/ (accessed 09 January 2024).

Health and Care Professions Council (2023a). Registrant Data and Statistics. Available: https://www.hcpc-uk.org/about-us/insights-and-data/the-register/ (accessed 09 January 2024).

Health and Care Professions Council (2023b). Registrant Snapshot – 1 March 2023. Available: https://www.hcpc-uk.org/resources/data/2023/registrant-snapshot-march-2023/ (accessed 09 January 2024).

Health and Care Professions Council (2023c). The Standards of Proficiency for Paramedics. Available: http://www.hcpc-uk.org/publications/standards/index.asp?id=48 (accessed 31 January 2024).

Health Education England. (2017). Multi-professional framework for advanced clinical practice in England. Available at: multi-professionalframeworkforadvancedclinicalpracticeinengland.pdf (hee.nhs.uk) (accessed 17 February 2024).

Health Education England. (2021). First Contact Practitioners and Advanced Practitioners in Primary Care: (Paramedic): A Roadmap to Practice. [Online]. Health Education England. Last Updated: January 2021. Available at: https://www.hee.nhs.uk/sites/default/files/documents/Paramedics-FINAL%20%28002%29.pdf (accessed 17 February 2024).

Health Foundation (2010). Ruling on Dr Andrew Wakefield in MMR Scare. Available: https://navigator.health.org.uk/theme/ruling-dr-andrew-wakefield-mmr-scare (accessed 09 January 2024).

Healthcare Services Safety Investigations Body (2020). Delayed Recognition of Acute Aortic Dissection. Available at: https://www.hssib.org.uk/patient-safety-investigations/delayed-recognition-of-acute-aortic-dissection/#:~:text=Acute%20aortic%20dissection%20is%20a%20relatively%20rare%20but,for%20other%20conditions%2C%20leading%20to%20delay%20in%20diagnosis (accessed 09 January 2024).

Healthcare Services Safety Investigations Body (2021a). Who We Are. Available: https://www.hsib.org.uk/about-us/ (accessed 09 January 2024).

Healthcare Services Safety Investigations Body (2021b). Residual Drugs in Cannulae and Extension Lines. Available: https://hsib-kqcco125-media.s3.amazonaws.com/staging-assets/documents/HSIB_Residual_drugs_in_intravenous_cannulae_and_extension_lines_Report_V07_kVFzcf9.pdf (accessed 09 January 2024).

Healthcare Services Safety Investigations Body (2021c). Never Events: Analysis of HSIB's National Investigations Report. Available: https://www.hsib.org.uk/documents/272/HSIB_Never_Events_-_analysis_of_HSIBs_national_investigations_Report_V09.pdf (accessed 09 January 2024).

Hicks, C. (1998). Barriers to evidence-based care in nursing: Historical legacies and conflicting cultures. *Health Services Management Research*, 11: 137–147.

Higginson, R., Jones, B., Kerr, T. and Ridley, A.M., (2020). Paramedic use of PPE and testing during the COVID-19 pandemic. *Journal of Paramedic Practice*, 12(6), pp. 221–225.

Higgs, J., Jones, M.A., Loftus, S. and Christensen, N. (2008). *Clinical Reasoning in the Health Professions*, 3rd edn. Oxford: Elsevier.

Hobbs, L., Devenish, S., Long, D. and Tippett, V., (2021). Facilitators, barriers and motivators of paramedic continuing professional development. *Australasian Journal of Paramedicine*, 18, pp. 1–7.

Hodge, A., Swift, S. and Wilson, J.P., (2018). Maintaining competency: a qualitative study of clinical supervision and mentorship as a framework for specialist paramedics. *British Paramedic Journal*, *3*(3), pp. 10–15.

Hodgett, R. and Ward, R., (2020). Are cervical collars effective and safe in prehospital spinal cord injury management?. *Journal of Paramedic Practice*, 12(2), pp. 67–78.

Höglund, E., Andersson-Hagiwara, M., Schröder, A., Möller, M. and Ohlsson-Nevo, E., (2020). Characteristics of non-conveyed patients in emergency medical services (EMS): a one-year prospective descriptive and comparative study in a region of Sweden. *BMC emergency medicine*, 20(1), pp. 1–11.

Holden, P.J., Carayon, P., Gurses, A.P., Hoonakker, P., Hundt A.S. et al. (2013). SEIPS 2.0: A human factors framework for studying and improving the work of healthcare professionals and patients. *Ergonomics*, 56(11): 1669–1686. Available: https://doi.org/10.1080/00140139.2013.838643 (accessed 09 January 2024).

Hollnagel, E., Wears, R.L. and Braithwaite, J. (2015). *From Safety-I to Safety-II: A White Paper. The Resilient Health Care Net.* Published simultaneously by the University of Southern Denmark, University of Florida, USA and Macquarie University, Australia.

Hopcroft, K. and Forte, V., (2020). *Symptom Sorter*. Abingdon: CRC Press.

Hope, T. (2004). *Medical Ethics: A Very Short Introduction*. Oxford: Oxford University Press.

Hughes, M., and Nimmo, G. (2016). Models of Clinical Reasoning. In Frain., J. and Cooper., N. (eds) *ABC of Clinical Reasoning*. Oxford: BMJ Books.

Hunt, P. (ed.) (2004). *International Companion Encyclopaedia of Children's Literature*. London: Routledge.

Hurwitz, B. (2004). How does evidence based guidance influence determinations of medical negligence? *BMJ Online*. Available: https://www.bmj.com/content/suppl/2004/10/28/329.7473.1024.DC1 (accessed 09 January 2024).

Ibarra, H. (1999). *Provisional Selves: Experimenting with Image and Identity in Professional Adaptation*. Available: http://dobweb.mit.edu/curhan/www/docs/Articles/15341_Readings/Self-presentation_Impression_Formation/Ibarra_1999_Provisional_selves.pdf (accessed 22 January 2024).

Iserson, K., Sanders, A., and Mathieu, D. (1995). *Ethics in Emergency Medicine*. Tuscon: Galen Press.

Jensen, J., Socha, D. (2013). *EMS Chiefs of Canada National Research Agenda*. Paramedic Chiefs of Canada.

Johnson, G. and Hill-Smith, I. (2006). *The Minor Illness Manual*. 4th edn. London: Radcliffe Publishing Ltd.

Joint Commission on Accreditation of Healthcare Organizations (2005). National Patient Safety Goals. Available: https://www.jointcommission.org/standards/national-patient-safety-goals/ (accessed 22 January 2024).

Jones, M., Butler, J., Graber, C.J. et al. (2017). Think twice: A cognitive perspective of an antibiotic timeout intervention to improve antibiotic use. *J Biomed Inform*, 71S: S22–31.

Kahneman, D. (2012). *Thinking Fast and Slow*. London: Penguin.

Kahneman, D. and Tversky, A. (1979). Prospect theory: An analysis of decision under risk. *Econometrica*, 47(2): 263–292. Available: https://doi.org/10.2307/1914185 (accessed 22 January 2024).

Kant, I. (2012). *Groundwork of the Metaphysics of Morals*. Gregor, M. and Timmerman, J. (eds), Cambridge: Cambridge University Press.

Kant, I. (trans. Bennett, J.) (2008). *Grounding for the Metaphysics of Morals*, 3rd edn. Indianapolis: Hackett.

Kassirer., J. Wong, J. and Kopelman., R. (2010). *Learning Clinical Reasoning*. Philadelphia: Lippincott Williams and Wilkins.

Khan, S. (2021). Cultural humility vs. cultural competence — and why providers need both. [Online]. Health City. Last Updated: March 2021. Available at: https://healthcity.bmc.org/policy-and-industry/cultural-humility-vs-cultural-competence-providers-ne [Accessed 18 February 2024].

King, I. and Clark, J.M. (2002). Intuition and the development of expertise in surgical ward and intensive care nurses. *Journal of Advanced Nursing*, 37(4): 322–329.

King's Fund. (2016). Long-term Conditions and Multi-morbidity. Available: www.kingsfund.org.uk/time-to-think-differently/trends/disease-and-disability/long-term-conditions-multi-morbidity (accessed 22 January 2024).

Kitchener, K.S., (1984). Intuition, critical evaluation and ethical principles: The foundation for ethical decisions in counseling psychology. *The counseling psychologist*, 12(3), pp. 43–55.

Klein, G.A., Orasanu, J.M. and Calderwood, R. (1993). *Decision Making in Action: Models and Methods*. Norwood, NJ: Ablex.

Kremer, M.J., Faut-Callahan, M. and Hicks, F.D. (2002). A study of clinical decision making by certified registered nurse anesthetists. *American Association of Nurse Anesthetists Journal*, 70(5): 391–397.

Lamond, D. and Thompson, C. (2000). Intuition and analysis in decision making and choice. *Journal of Nursing Scholarship*, 32(3): 411–414.

Larkin, J., McDermott, J., Simon, O.P. and Simon, H.A. (1980). Expert and novice performance in solving physics problems. *Science*, 208(4450): 1335–1342.

Leaper, C. (2011). Self-categorization (and social identity) theory. Available: https://www.sciencedirect.com/topics/psychology/social-identity-theory (accessed 22 January 2024).

Leonard, M., Graham, S. and Bonacum, D. (2004). The human factor: The critical importance of effective teamwork and communication in providing safe care. *Quality & Safety in Health Care* 13(Suppl 1): i85–i90.

Levac, L., McMurtry, L., Stienstra, D., Baikie, G., Hanson, C., Mucina, D., (2018). Learning across Indigenous and Western knowledge systems and intersectionality: Reconciling social science research approaches. University of Guelph. Available: https://www.criaw-icref.ca/wp-content/uploads/2021/04/Learning-Across-Indigenous-and-Western-KnowledgesFINAL.pdf (accessed 29 April 2026).

Light, D.W., 2010. Health-care professions, markets and countervailing powers. In: Bird, C., Conrad, P., Fremont, A., and Timmermans, S. (eds) *Handbook of medical sociology,* 6(1), pp. 270–289.

Lockey, D.J., Healey, B., Crewdson, K., Chalk, G., Weaver, A.E. and Davies, G.E., (2015). Advanced airway management is necessary in prehospital trauma patients. *British journal of anaesthesia*, 114(4), pp. 657–662.

Lopez, J. (2020). Unconscious bias training. Available: https://questions-statements.parliament.uk/written-statements/detail/2020-12-15/hcws652 (accessed 22 January 2024).

Lord, B. and Khalsa, S. (2019). Influence of patient race on administration of analgesia by student paramedics. *BMC Emergency Medicine*, 19(32). Available: https://bmcemergmed.biomedcentral.com/articles/10.1186/s12873-019-0245-2 (assessed 22 April 2026).

Lovegrove, M. and Davis, J. (2013). *Paramedic Evidence Based Education Project (PEEP).* Bridgwater: College of Paramedics.

Madden, N. (2018). Graded Assertiveness: Captain, I Have a Concern.... *gCaptain*. Available: https://gcaptain.com/graded-assertiveness-captain-i-have-a-concern/ (accessed 22 January 2024).

Mahase, E. (2020). Black babies are less likely to die when cared for by black doctors, US study finds. *British Medical Journal*, 370. Available: https://www.bmj.com/content/370/bmj.m3315_ (accessed 22 January 2024).

Majchrowska, A., Pawlikowski, J., Jojczuk, M., Nogalski, A., Bogusz, R., Nowakowska, L. and Wiechetek, M., (2021). Social prestige of the paramedic profession. *International Journal of Environmental Research and Public Health*, 18(4), p. 1506.

Manias, E. and Street, A. (2001). Nurses and doctors communicating through medication order charts in critical care. *Australian Critical Care*, 14(1): 17–23.

Martin, A.C. and O'Meara, P. (2019). Perspectives from the frontline of two North American community paramedicine programs: An observational, ethnographic study. *Rural and Remote Health*, 19(1): 71–79.

Martinez, R., Rogers, A.D., Numanoglu, A. and Rode, H. (2018). The value of WhatsApp communication in paediatric burn care. *Burns: Journal of the International Society for Burn Injuries*, 44(4): 947–955.

Martín-Rodríguez, F., López-Izquierdo, R., del Pozo Vegas, C., Benito, J.F.D., Rodríguez, V.C., Rasilla, M.N.D., Conty, J.L.M., Iscar, A.M., de la Torre, S.O., Martín, V.M. and Villamor, M.A.C., (2019). Accuracy of national early warning score 2 (NEWS2) in prehospital triage on in-hospital early *mortality: a multi-center observational prospective cohort study. Prehospital and disaster medicine*, 34(6), pp. 610–618.

MBRRACE (Mothers and Babies: Reducing Risk through Audit and Confidential Enquiry). (2019). *Saving Lives, Improving Mothers' Care*. Oxford: MBRRACE/University of Oxford.

Meek, J., Stewart, R., (2024). Treat them where they lie, Pioneering a revolution in modern emergency medicine. Halifax: Nimbus Publishing Limited.

Mehrabian, A. (1981). Silent messages: Implicit communication of emotions and attitudes. Belmont, CA: Wadsworth. Available: https://www.businessballs.com/communication-skills/mehrabians-communication-theory-verbal-non-verbal-body-language/ (accessed 22 January 2024).

Miles, J., Coster, J. and Jacques, R., (2019). Using vignettes to assess the accuracy and rationale of paramedic decisions on conveyance to the emergency department. *British Paramedic Journal*, 4(1), pp. 6–13.

Mill, J.S. (1989). *On Liberty and Other Writings*. Collini, S. (ed.). Cambridge: Cambridge University Press.

Ministry of Housing, Communities & Local Government (2019). *The English Indices of Deprivation 2019 (IoD2019)*. Available: https://assets.publishing.service.gov.uk/government/uploads/system/uploads/attachment_data/file/835115/IoD2019_Statistical_Release.pdf (accessed 09 January 2024).

Muir, N. (2004). Clinical decision making: Theory and practice. *Nursing Standard*, 18(36): 47–52.

Murdoch, I. (1971). *The Sovereignty of Good*. London: Routledge.

MUSC (Medical University of South Carolina). (n.d.). Kenneth Catchpole PhD. Available: https://education.musc.edu/MUSCApps/facultydirectory/Catchpole-Kenneth (accessed 22 January 2024).

National Institute for Health and Care Excellence (NICE). (2024). Spinal injury: assessment and Initial management. Available at: https://www.nice.org.uk/guidance/ng41/chapter/recommendations (accessed February 2024).

Newton, A., Hunt, B. and Williams, J. (2020). The paramedic profession: Disruptive innovation and barriers to further progress. *Journal of Paramedic Practice*, 12(4): 138–148.

NHS Digital. (2014). National Statistics Ambulance Services, England 2013–14. Available: https://digital.nhs.uk/data-and-information/publications/statistical/ambulance-services/ambulance-services-england-2013-14 (accessed 22 January 2024).

NHS England & Public Health England. (2016). Making Every Contact Count (MECC): Consensus statement. [Online]. NHS England. Last Updated: 2016. Available at: https://www.england.nhs.uk/wp-content/uploads/2016/04/making-every-contact-count.pdf [accessed 18 February 2024].

NHS England (2013). Transforming Urgent and Emergency Care Services in England. Urgent and Emergency Care Review, End of Phase 1 Report. Available: www.nhs.uk/NHSEngland/keogh-review/Documents/UECR.Ph1Report.FV.pdf (accessed 22 January 2024).

NHS England. (2014a) The 6 Cs. Available: https://www.healthcareers.nhs.uk/about/working-health/6cs. Last accessed November 2016.

NHS England. (2014b). The Five Year Forward View. Available: www.england.nhs.uk/wp-content/uploads/2014/10/5yfv-web.pdf (accessed 22 January 2024).

NHS England. (2016). Confidentiality Policy. Available: https://www.england.nhs.uk/wp-content/uploads/2019/10/confidentiality-policy-v5.1.pdf (accessed 22 January 2024).

NHS England. (2019a). Breaking down barriers to better health and care. Available: https://www.england.nhs.uk/publication/breaking-down-barriers-to-better-health-and-care/ (accessed 23 January 2024).

NHS England. (2019b). Shared Decision-Making: Summary Guide. Available at: https://www.england.nhs.uk/publication/shared-decision-making-summary-guide/ (accessed 23 January 2024).

NHS England. (2021). Ambulance Quality Indicators. Available: https://www.england.nhs.uk/statistics/statistical-work-areas/ambulance-quality-indicators/ (accessed 23 January 2024).

NHS England. (2022). Agenda for Change. Available: https://www.healthcareers.nhs.uk/working-health/working-nhs/nhs-pay-and-benefits/agenda-change-pay-rates/agenda-change-pay-rates (accessed 23 January 2024).

NHS England. (n.d.a). Shared professional decision-making: Putting collective leadership into practice. Available: https://www.england.nhs.uk/nursingmidwifery/shared-governance-and-collective-leadership/sdm/ (accessed 23 January 2024).

NHS England. (n.d.b). Enhancing the quality of life for people living with long term conditions. Available: https://www.england.nhs.uk/wp-content/uploads/2014/09/ltc-infographic.pdf (accessed 23 January 2024).

NHS Professionals. (n.d.). The 6 Cs of Care. [Online]. NHS Professionals. Last Updated: n.d.. Available at: https://www.nhsprofessionals.nhs.uk/nhs-staffing-pool-hub/working-in-healthcare/the-6-cs-of-care [Accessed 18 February 2024].

Nicol J., Nyatanga B. (2017). *Palliative and end of life care in nursing* (2nd edn.). London, UK: SAGE Publications Limited.

Nik Muhamad, N.A. (2019). Confidence level and knowledge of pre-hospital thrombolysis therapy of paramedic in pre-hospital care: A survey. *Medicine and Health*, 14(1): 34–43.

Noddings, N. and Shore, P.J. (1984). *Awakening the Inner Eye: Intuition in Education*. London: Teachers College Press.

Nordby, H. and Nøhr, Ø. (2012). The ethics of resuscitation: How do paramedics experience ethical dilemmas when faced with cancer patients with cardiac arrest? *Prehospital and Disaster Medicine*, 27(1): 64–70.

Norman, D. (2013). *The Design of Everyday Things*. New York: Basic Books.

NSRoP (2025). Nova Scotia Regulator of Paramedicine. Available: https://www.nsrop.ca/9accessed 10 April 2026).

O'Hara, R., Johnson, M., Siriwardena, A.N., Weyman, A., Turner, J., Shaw, D., Mortimer, P., Newman, C., Hirst, E., Storey, M. and Mason, S., (2015). A qualitative study of systemic influences on paramedic decision making: care transitions and patient safety. *Journal of health services research & policy*, *20*(1_suppl), pp. 45–53.

O'Sullivan, E.D. (2018). Cognitive bias in clinical medicine. *Journal of the Royal College of Physicians Edinburgh*, 48: 225–232. Available: http://www.rcpe.ac.uk/sites/default/files/jrcpe_48_3_osullivan.pdf (accessed 23 January 2024).

O'Sullivan, J.W., Albasri, A., Nicholson, B.D. et al. (2018). Overtesting and undertesting in primary care: A systematic review and meta-analysis. BMJ Open, 8(2). Available: https://bmjopen.bmj.com/content/8/2/e018557 (accessed 09 January 2024).

Oboro, V., Akinmoladun, J., Oboro, O., Isawumi, A., Awopetu, O. and Adelakun, I. (2015). P13.01: Reproducibility of fetal biometry by an inexperienced paramedic using both two- and three-dimensional ultrasound. *Ultrasound in Obstetrics & Gynecology*, 46: 161.

O'Cathain, A., Knowles, E., Bishop-Edwards, L., Coster, J., Crum, A. et al. (2018). Understanding variation in ambulance service non-conveyance rates: A mixed methods study. *Health Services and Delivery Research*, May.

Office for National Statistics (ONS) (2018). National population projections: 2018-based. Available: https://www.ons.gov.uk/peoplepopulationandcommunity/populationandmigration/populationprojections/bulletins/nationalpopulationprojections/2018based (accessed 23 January 2024).

Office for National Statistics (ONS) (2021). National population projections: 2020-based interim. Available: https://www.ons.gov.uk/peoplepopulationandcommunity/populationandmigration/populationprojections/bulletins/nationalpopulationprojections/2020basedinterim (accessed 23 January 2024).

Office for National Statistics (ONS) (2022). National population projections: 2020-based interim. Available: https://www.ons.gov.uk/peoplepopulationandcommunity/populationandmigration/populationprojections/bulletins/nationalpopulationprojections/2020basedinterim (accessed 23 January 2024).

Offredy, M. (1998). The application of decision making concepts by nurse practitioners in primary care. *Journal of Advanced Nursing*, 40: 988–1000.

Oxford English Dictionary (OED) (2013). Available: http://www.oed.com/ (accessed 23 January 2024).

Paris Jr, J.F. (2014). *Lessons from Mount Stupid*. Available: https://opexsociety.org/body-of-knowledge/lessons-from-mount-stupid/ (accessed 23 January 2024).

Patel, V.L. and Groen, G.J. (1986). Knowledge based solution strategies in medical reasoning. *Cognitive Science*, 10: 91–116.

Paul, R. and Elder, L. (2001). *Miniature Guide to Critical Thinking*. Tomales: Foundation for Critical Thinking.

Pertwee, E., Simas, C. and Larson, H.J. (2022). An epidemic of uncertainty: Rumors, conspiracy theories and vaccine hesitancy. *Nature Medicine*, 28: 456–459. Available: https://www.nature.com/articles/s41591-022-01728-z (accessed 23 January 2024).

PHEM Feedback (2023). Learning from patients, for patients. Available: https://www.phemfeedback.org/index.php (accessed 23 January 2024).

Philips, L. and Rempushki, V. (1985). A decision making model for diagnosing and intervening in elder abuse and neglect. *Nursing Research*, 34(3): 134–139.

Phillips, J.S., (2020). Paramedics' perceptions and experiences of NHS 111 in the south west of England. *Journal of Paramedic Practice*, 12(6), pp. 227–234.

Pirolli, P. and Card, S., (2005). The sensemaking process and leverage points for analyst technology as identified through cognitive task analysis. In *Proceedings of international conference on intelligence analysis* (Vol. 5, pp. 2–4).

Pollard, J. and Black, S. (2015). Do paramedics find it beneficial to learn the diagnosis given to their patients in the emergency department? *Emergency Medicine Journal*. [e-journal] 32:421. http://dx.doi.org/10.1136/emermed-2015-204877.2

Prichard, H.A. (1949). *Moral Obligation*. Oxford: Oxford University Press.

PPAO (Professional Paramedic Association Ottawa) (2026). *History of Paramedicine*. Available https://www.ottawaparamedics.ca/Before-9-1-1/history-of-paramedicine9 (accessed 27 February 2026).

Project Implicit. (2011). Project Implicit. [Online]. Project Implicit. Available at: https://www.projectimplicit.net/ (accessed 09 March 2024).

Province of Nova Scotia (2025). Regulated Health Professions Act Chapter 15 of the ACTS of 2023. Authority of the Speaker of the House of Assembly Halifax, Nova Scotia, Canada.

Public Health England (2018). Health profile for England: 2018. Chapter 3: trends in morbidity and risk factors. Available: https://www.gov.uk/government/publications/health-profile-for-england-2018/chapter-3-trends-in-morbidity-and-risk-factors (accessed 23 January 2024).

Pyles, S. and Stern, P. (1983). Discovery of nursing gestalt in critical care nursing: The importance of the Grey Gorilla Syndrome image. *Journal of Nursing Scholarship*, XV(2): 51–52.

Radcliffe, J. and Heath, G., (2009). Ambulance calls and cancellations: policy and implementation issues. *International Journal of Public Sector Management*, *22*(5), pp. 410–422.

Radwin, L.E. (1990). Research on diagnostic reasoning in nursing. *Nursing Diagnosis*, 1(2): 70–77.

Ragau, S., Hitchcock, R., Craft, J. and Christensen, M. (2018). Using the HALT model in an exploratory quality improvement initiative to reduce medication errors. *British Journal of Nursing*, 27(22). Available: https://www.magonlinelibrary.com/doi/abs/10.12968/bjon.2018.27.22.1330 (accessed 09 January 2024).

Rawls, J. (1971). *A Theory of Justice*. Cambridge, MA: Harvard University Press.

Reason, J. (1997). *Managing the Risks of Organizational Accidents*. London: Routledge.

Reed, M.J., Gibson, L., Dewar, A., Short, S., Black, P. and Clegg, G.R. (2017). Introduction of paramedic led Echo in Life Support into the pre-hospital environment: The PUCA study. *Resuscitation*, 112: 65–69.

Rees, N., Smythe, L., Hogan, C. and Williams, J. (2021). Paramedic experiences of providing care in Wales (UK) during the 2020 COVID-19 pandemic (PECC-19): a qualitative study using evolved grounded theory. *BMJ open*, 11(6), p.e048677.

Rew, L. (1986). Intuition concept analysis of a group phenomenon. *Advances in Nursing Science*, 8(2): 21–28.

Rimoldi, H. (1988). Diagnosing the diagnostic process. *Medical Education*, 22(4): 270–278.

Riskin, A., Erez, A., Foulk, T.A. et al. (2015). The impact of rudeness on medical team performance: A randomized trial. *Paediatrics*, 136(3): 487–495.

RHP Act (2024). The Regulated Health Professions Act. Available here: https://nslegislature.ca/sites/default/files/legc/statutes/regulated%20health%20professions.pdf (accessed 10 April 2026).

Rock, D. and Grant, H. (2016). Why diverse teams are smarter. *Harvard Business Review*. Available: https://hbr.org/2016/11/why-diverse-teams-are-smarter (accessed 23 January 2024).

Rosenorn-Lanng, D. (2014). *Human Factors in Healthcare*. Oxford: Oxford University Press.

Ross, L., Boyle, M., Williams, B. et al. (2014). Perceptions of student paramedic interpersonal communication competence: A cross-sectional study. *Australian Journal of Paramedicine*, 11(4): 1–5.

Ross, W.D. (2002). *The Right and The Good.* New York: OUP.

Runzheimer, J. and Johnson Larsen, L. (2011). *Medical Ethics for Dummies*. Hoboken, NJ: Wiley.

Rutherford, G. (2020). *Human Factors in Paramedic Practice*. Bridgwater: Class Professional Publishing.

St Francis Xavier University, (2009). Diploma in Adult Education, Module 2, Learning Objectives Readings and Appendices.

Scanlon, T.M. (1998). *What We Owe to Each Other*. Cambridge, MA: Harvard University Press.

Schaeffer, J. (1974). The interrelatedness of decision making and the nursing process. *American Journal of Nursing*, 74(10): 1852–1855.

Schon, D. (1983). *The Reflective Practitioner: How Professionals Think in Action*. London: Temple Smith.

Scott, J., (2020). Re-contact rates with a UK ambulance service following paramedic referral to a falls prevention service for those aged≥ 65 years: a retrospective cohort study. *British paramedic journal*, *5*(2), pp. 18–25.

Simon, C., Everitt, H. and Kendrick, T. (2005). *Oxford Handbook of General Practice*. Oxford: Oxford University Press.

Simons, D. (2010). The Monkey Business Illusion. Available: www.dansimons.com/videos.html (accessed 23 January 2024).

Sommers, N., Evans, L., Collingwood, T. et al. (2019). PP29 'Breaking down Barriers': Experiences from the first year of an ED to EMS feedback 'Postbox'. *Emergency Medicine Journal*, 36(10): e13.

Standing, M. (2008). Clinical judgement and decision making in nursing – nine modes of practice in a revised cognitive continuum. *Journal of Advanced Nursing*, 62(1): 124–134.

Standing, M. (2017). *Clinical Judgement and Decision Making for Nursing Students*, 3rd edn. London: Learning Matters (Sage).

Steventon, A., Deeny, S., Friebel, R., Gardner, T., Thorlby, R. (2018). *Briefing: Emergency Hospital Admissions in England: Which May Be Avoidable and How?* London: The Health Foundation.

Sullivan, E.J. and Decker, P.J. (2003). *Effective Leadership and Management in Nursing*. London: Pearson Prentice Hall.

Syed, M. (2011). *Bounce: The Myth of Talent and the Power of Practice*. New York: Fourth Estate.

Tajfel, H. and Turner, J.C. (1979). An integrative theory of intergroup conflict. In: Austin, W.G. and Worchel, S. (eds). *The Social Psychology of Intergroup Relations*. Monterey, CA: Brooks/Cole, pp. 33–37.

Tang, S., Brady, M., Mildenhall, J., Rolfe, U., Bowles, A. and Morgan, K., (2020). The new coronavirus disease: what do we know so far? *Journal of Paramedic Practice*, 12(5), pp. 193–201.

Tavares. W., Allana. A., Beaune, L., Weiss, D., and Blanchard, I. (2022). Principles to Guide the Future of Paramedicine in Canada, *Prehospital Emergency Care*, 26(5): 728–738.

Thompson, C. (1999). A conceptual treadmill: The need for 'middle ground' in clinical decision making theory in nursing. *Journal of Advanced Nursing*, 30(5): 1222–1229.

Thompson, C. and Dowding, D. (2002). *Decision Making and Judgement in Nursing – An Introduction*. Philadelphia, PN: Churchill Livingstone.

Torabi, M., Borhani, F., Abbaszadeh, A. and Atashzadeh-Shoorideh, F. (2019). Ethical decision-making based on field assessment: The experiences of prehospital personnel. *Nursing Ethics*, 26(4), 1075–1086.

Townsend, R. (2017). The role of the law in the professionalisation of paramedicine in Australia. Doctoral Thesis, Australian National University.

Truth and Reconciliation Commission of Canada: Calls to Action (2012). Truth and Reconciliation Commission of Canada

Turner, J. and Williams, J. (2018). An evaluation of early stage development of rotating paramedic model pilot sites. Available at: https://uhra.herts.ac.uk/bitstream/handle/2299/21174/Rotating_Paramedics_Final_Report.pdf (accessed February 2024).

Tversky, A. and Kahneman, D. (1974). Judgment under uncertainty: Heuristics and biases. *Science*, 185: 1124–1131.

Tversky, A. and Kahneman, D. (1982). Judgments of and by representativeness. In: Kahneman, D., Slovic, P. and Tversky, A. (eds). *Judgment Under Uncertainty: Heuristics and Biases.* Cambridge: Cambridge University Press.

Tversky, A., and Kahneman, D. (1983). Extensional Versus Intuitive reasoning: The Conjunction Fallacy in Probability Judgment, *Psychol. Rev*, 90(4). doi: 10.1037/0033-295X.90.4.293.

Ubel, P.A., Scherr, K.A. and Fagerlin, A., (2017). Empowerment failure: how shortcomings in physician communication unwittingly undermine patient autonomy. *The American Journal of Bioethics*, 17(11), pp. 31–39.

UK Government (2015). 2010 to 2015 government policy: Long term health conditions. Available: https://www.gov.uk/government/publications/2010-to-2015-government-policy-long-term-health-conditions/2010-to-2015-government-policy-long-term-health-conditions (accessed 23 January 2024).

UK Government (2018). *Data Protection Act.* Available: https://www.legislation.gov.uk/ukpga/2018/12/contents/enacted (accessed 23 January 2024).

UK Government. (2023). Reported road casualties in Great Britain, provisional estimates: year ending June 2023. [Online]. UK Government. Last Updated: November 2023. Available at: Reported road casualties in Great Britain, provisional estimates: year ending June 2023 - GOV.UK. Available: https://www.gov.uk/government/statistics/reported-road-casualties-in-great-britain-provisional-estimates-year-ending-june-2023/reported-road-casualties-in-great-britain-provisional-estimates-year-ending-june-2023 (accessed 17 February 2024).

UK Sepsis Trust (2024). *Sepsis.* Available: http://sepsistrust.org/professional/help-my-organisation/ https://sepsistrust.org/professional-resources/ (accessed 27 February 2024).

University of Ottawa (2026). In Memoriam: Dr. Justin Maloney. Available at: https://www.uottawa.ca/faculty-medicine/news/memoriam-dr-justin-maloney (accessed 02 March 2026).

van der Gaag, A., Jago, R., Austin, Z., Zasada, M., Banks, S., Gallagher, A. and Lucas, G. (2018). Why do paramedics have a high rate of self-referral? *Journal of Paramedic Practice*, *10*(5), pp. 205–210.

van Dongen, D.N., Ottervanger, J.P., Tolsma, R., Fokkert, M., van der Sluis, A., van 't Hof, A.W., Badings, E. and Slingerland, R.J. (2019). In-hospital healthcare utilization, outcomes, and costs in pre-hospital-adjudicated low-risk chest-pain patients. *Applied Health Economics and Health Policy*, 17, pp. 875–882.

Vincent, C. & Taylor-Adams, S. (2001). The investigation and analysis of clinical incidents. In: Vincent, C. (ed.), *Clinical Risk Management: Enhacning Patient Safety*. London: BMJ Books, pp. 439–460.

Weick, K. E. (2005). The experience of theorizing: Sensemaking as topic and resource. In K. G. Smith and M. A. Hitt (Eds), *Great Minds in Management: The Process of Theory Development*. Oxford: Oxford University Press, 394–413.

Weick, K.E. (1995). *Sensemaking in Organizations*. Thousand Oaks, CA: Sage.

Weick, K.E., Kathleen, M. and Sutcliffe, K.M. (2015). *Managing the Unexpected Sustained Performance in a Complex World* (3rd edn). Hoboken, NJ: Wiley.

Welsh, I. and Lyons, C.M. (2001). Evidence-based care and the case for intuitive and tacit knowledge in clinical assessment and decision making in mental health nursing practice: An empirical contribution to the debate. *Journal of Psychiatric and Mental Health Nursing*, 8: 299–305.

Winters, B.D., Gurses, A.P., Lehmann, H., Sexton, J.B., Rampersad, C.J. and Pronovost, P.J. (2009). Clinical review checklist – translating evidence into practice. *Critical Care*, 13(210): 2.

Woollard, M., O'Meara, P. and Munro, G. (2010). What price 90 seconds: Is 'Call Connect' a disservice to 999 callers? *Emergency Medical Journal*, 27: 729–730.

World Health Organization (WHO) (2008). WHO Surgical Safety Checklist and Implementation Manual. Available: https://www.who.int/publications/i/item/9789241598590 (accessed 23 January 2024).

World Health Organization (WHO) (2009). Surgical Safety Checklist. Available: https://apps.who.int/iris/bitstream/handle/10665/44186/9789241598590_eng_Checklist.pdf;jsessionid=DA (accessed 23 January 2024).

Yeager, K.A., and Bauer-Wu, S. (2013). Cultural humility: essential foundation for clinical researchers. *Applied Nursing Research: ANR*, 26(4), 251–256.

Yudkowsky, E.S. (2003). An intuitive explanation of Bayes' Theorem. Available: http://yudkowsky.net/rational/bayes (accessed 23 January 2024).

Zimbardo, P.G., Haney, C., Banks, W.C. and Jaffe, D. (1971). *The Stanford Prison Experiment*. Zimbardo, Incorporated.

Index

A

Aboriginal communities, 91
  see also Indigenous populations
abdominal pain, 66, 75, 76, 115, 116, 143, 164, 185–9
abductive reasoning, 53–4, 134
absolutism, 123t
action bias, 76–7, 193
active listening, 96
acuity, 1, 9–10, 22, 39, 60, 62, 131, 145, 165, 176–7, 199
acumen, 15, 17, 68, 79, 107, 112, 134, 151, 199
acute coronary syndrome, 174
advocacy, 1, 3, 25
age, 11
agency, 29, 88, 199
Air Accident Investigation Branch (AAIB), 67
alcohol, 32, 52–4, 148, 168, 170
allied health professionals (AHPs), 7, 199
allyship, 88–90, 89fig
ambulance resource problem, 37–8, 38fig
anaemia, 100
analytical reasoning, 126fig
anchoring bias, 71, 159
anterior ST segment elevation, 152, 199
anticoagulant therapy, 176–82
anxiety, 8, 16, 67, 72, 105, 109, 134, 152, 158–9, 169, 191
Apixaban, 176, 178, 179
appendicitis, 76, 115, 164, 187
The Art of Thinking Clearly, 73
association bias, 87, 117, 169, 171, 173, 175, 177, 179
asthma, 185
atrial fibrillation, 176, 178
authority bias, 74, 177, 181, 193, 195, 199
autonomy, 12, 18, 21–5, 29–37, 34fig, 39, 41, 43, 79, 145, 152, 199
availability bias, 72, 149, 158, 159, 169, 173, 177, 179
averages bias, 77–8, 190, 191
aviation, 74, 114, 118, 120–21

B

base-rate neglect, 75–199
beneficence, 28–31, 34fig, 36–7, 39–41, 152, 199
biases, 70–78, 84–8, 90–93, 100, 104, 118–19, 149, 158, 193
  conscious, 86–8
  decision making and, 87–90
  defined, 82, 84
  in-groups and out-groups, 85
  paramedics and, 88, 91
  reasons for, 86–8
  System 1 and System 2 thinking, 58–9
  unconscious, 86–8
bioethics, 15, 26–27, 31, 41, 43, 47, 108
  beneficence, 28–31, 34fig, 36–7, 39–41, 152, 199
  ethical decision making in paramedic practice, 31–2
  justice, 28–30, 36–7, 39, 41, 43, 47, 67–8, 73, 75, 152, 171, 184, 194
  means to an end, 6, 33, 42–3, 179
  non-maleficence, 28, 30, 35–6, 39, 152, 171, 184, 194
  overview of, 26–7, 31, 41, 43, 47
  paramedic ethical decision-making model, 40–41, 41fig
  professionalism and, 43, 47
  respect for autonomy, 29, 34, 36, 39, 41
  see also ethics
blood
  glucose, 76, 150
  pressure, 72, 103, 113, 144, 149–50
  tests, 135, 145, 150–51
Bolam test, 162
brain injury, 178–9
Bromiley, Martin, 61, 74, 163
bruising, 100

C

Canadian Organization of Paramedic Regulators (COPR), 4, 5, 17, 33, 47, 82
Canadian Paramedic Competency Framework (CPCF), 5, 33, 82, 175
capability line, 144fig, 170, 175
car accidents, 154
cardiac arrest, 19, 27, 37, 54, 60, 77, 92, 125, 139, 165, 175, 182
see also heart attacks; myocardial infarction

Cardiopulmonary Resuscitation (CPR), 29, 39, 76, 130, 169, 173, 182
see also resuscitation
career
Career Framework, 4, 6–7, 8fig
development, 4–8
guidance, 4–8
care provision, 2
case studies
autonomy, 29–37
decision making, 168, 172, 176, 180, 185, 189, 192
female, car crash 189–92
female with abdominal pain, 185–9
female with headache, 168–72
female with head injury on anticoagulant therapy, 176–180
female with respiratory illness, 180–85
hypothetico-deductive model, 55–6
information processing, 113–16
male with GI bleed 192–6
male with productive cough and chest pain, 172–5
structure, 167–8
causal reasoning, 54
caution, 107
change, 124t
Charlin, B., 143
checklists, 49, 56, 69–70, 114, 121
chest
infection, 172–6
pain, 172–5
choking, 77
chronic obstructive pulmonary disease (COPD), 54
Clinical Human Factors Group, 61, 69
close-mindedness, 124t
clotting, 179
see also anticoagulant therapy; novel anticoagulant drugs (NOACs)
cockpit resource management (CRM), 74
cognition, 58, 61, 134
cognitive continuum, 49, 61, 133–5, 142, 145
cognitive dissonance, 68, 123t
coital headaches, 169–70
collaborative decision making, 112, 147, 159
coma, 169, 178
comfort zones, 123t
communication, 69–70, 93–5, 131, 186
awareness, improving, 98
challenges to, 98–99t
elements of, 94
importance of, 97
language and vocabulary, 95
social and cultural context, 97–8
verbal, 95–6
written, 97
co-morbid, 8, 163
competency, 2–6, 12, 15, 18–19, 44–5, 75, 82–83, 90–91, 98, 115, 133–4, 136, 138–40, 145, 171, 175, 180, 186, 188, 197
competency frameworks, 3–4, 82, 91
complaints, 20, 55, 72, 100
complexity, 1, 9–10, 23, 32, 88, 95, 145
conditions of practice, 8, 11, 17, 19
conduct, 5, 57
confidence, 6, 8, 11–12, 15–16, 36, 44–5, 47, 75, 134, 136–7, 171
see also overconfidence bias
confidentiality, 15, 17, 28, 43, 197
confirmation bias, 74, 149, 151, 158, 177, 200
conformism, 123t
conjunction bias, 72–3, 186, 200
conscious bias, 86–8, 100, 105
conscious competence, 139t
conscious incompetence, 45, 139t
consent, 33, 42, 153, 156, 186
contagion bias, 78
continuous professional development (CPD), 18, 44, 67, 137, 152
contractualism, 28,36
conveyance rates, 77
COPD (chronic obstructive pulmonary disease), 54
COPR see Canadian Organization of Paramedic Regulators
coronary artery, 173
cough, 74, 142, 172–3, 181
CPD (continuous professional development), 10, 16, 55, 79, 158
CPCF see Canadian Paramedic Competency Framework
CPR (Cardiopulmonary Resuscitation), 29, 39, 76, 130, 169, 173, 182
see also resuscitation
crew resource management, 74
crime, 43, 199
critical care, 3, 12, 18, 22–4, 39, 41, 50, 59, 70
critical care specialty, 18
critical thinking
barriers to, 119–20, 122–5, 129, 131
breaking down, 119–20
decision point management, 107, 126–7
in everyday life, 108–10

intuition and experience in, 125, 126fig
value-based decision making and healthcare practice, 110–13
CRM (cockpit resource management), 74
CT scan, 53, 145, 151, 171
see also imaging
cultural competency, 82, 90–91
cultural humility, 82, 90–91
culture,44–5, 49, 61, 63–4, 67–9, 79, 81, 86, 89–90, 93, 100, 108–9, 124, 148, 158
curriculum, , 2, 7, 12, 88
cyanosis, 100

D

death and end of life care, 8, 101
decision making, shared, 33, 42, 145, 160, 195
decision point management, 107, 126–7, 167, 171
deductive reasoning, 51–2, 51fig, 55, 139, 170, 174, 179, 184, 188, 191, 194
see also hypothetico-deduction
defensible practice, 157
defensive practice, 157
dementia, 10, 29, 32, 60, 95
demography, 8, 78
denial, 116, 122–3, 123t, 189
deontology, 27–8, 41
deprivation, 9, 11–12
descriptive decision theory, 50
DH (drug history), 167, 169, 172, 176, 178, 181, 185, 190, 192
diabetes, 8, 11, 52, 149, 199
diagnosis, 21, 42, 44, 51, 54–5, 58, 74, 76, 81, 113, 116–17, 127, 130–1, 134, 143, 149, 151–3, 155, 158–9, 166, 168, 170–5, 181–6, 197
see also differential diagnoses
diagnostic reasoning, 115
differential diagnoses, 76, 127, 149, 158, 170, 174, 179, 183, 187, 194
dignity, 15, 29, 31, 35, 83
discernment, 124t
distractions,70–1, 79, 121, 173, 191
diversity, 81, 83, 92, 125
encouraging, 92–3
Dobelli, Rolf, 73, 78–9
doctrine of double effect, 35–6
documentation, 147, 154–7, 162, 165–6, 197
doubt, 57, 77
Dreyfus Model, 121, 133, 138–40
dual process theory, 49, 58, 60–1
Dunning-Kruger Effect, 1121, 136–7, 136fig
duty of care, 28

E

ECG, 52, 57fig, 105, 144, 149, 151–2, 174–5
ectopic pregnancy, 186, 188
education, 3–8, 12, 19, 21, 23–6, 33, 81–3, 88, 91–2, 101, 149, 178, 191
egocentrism, innate, 119t, 174
egotism, 120
Elder, Linda, 118
emergency care, 7, 21–2, 24, 26, 42, 72, 101, 171
emotional influence, 122, 123t
emotions, 33, 46, 51, 58, 96, 122
encephalitis, 170
end of life care, 8, 101
endotracheal intubation (ETI), 18
epidemiology, 8–9
epistemological self-confidence, 45
equality, 28, 30, 81, 86
equipment, 1–2, 21, 37, 70, 137, 161, 170
ergonomics, 61, 158
errors, 16, 46–7, 52, 56, 61, 64–8, 65fig, 70, 97, 114, 121, 125, 129t, 131, 134, 148, 152, 155
ethical decision making in paramedic practice, 31
ethics, 3, 17, 26–28, 30–1, 33, 40, 42, 46–7, 50, 67, 108, 152, 199
see also bioethics
ethnicity, 81, 85–6, 100
ethnocentrism, 124t
evidence-based medicine, 111
experience, 74, 125, 134, 136, 138, 140, 143, 149
experiential decision making, 75
expertise, 7, 22, 36, 43, 49, 63, 90, 117, 125, 133, 138t, 161
extended generalists, 188
extradural haemorrhage, 178

F

face-saving, 124t
failure, 11, 19, 62, 64, 75, 94, 119t, 120, 174
fallacies, 45, 70–1, 73–4, 119, 154, 169, 173, 177, 181–2, 186, 190
see also biases
falls, 10–11, 126–7, 165, 182
false causality bias, 76, 186
fatigue, 20, 46, 69, 169, 171
fear, 123–4t
feature-positive effect, 186
feedback, 50, 95, 100, 147, 152–3, 166, 191
feelings, 90, 96, 119t, 123t, 140
fever, 56, 74, 164, 172–3, 175, 181, 185
fitness to practise (FTP), 19, 86
fractures, 29, 149, 151, 157, 179, 191
fragility fracture, 11

First Nations, 101
Freidson's theory, 31, 35, 37
From Novice to Expert, 127, 144–5, 151, 155
FTP (fitness to practise), 20–1, 23, 25

G

Garden Gate Test, 133–19, 141–17, 195
Gardner, Dan, 154
gatekeeping, 16, 36
generalists, 7, 188
glucose levels, blood, 76, 150
GMC (General Medical Council), 24
groupthink, 108–10, 121, 124t, 182
  see also innate sociocentrism
gut feelings, 123t

H

haematoma, 176, 178–9
HALT mnemonic, 158
headache, 1168–72, 176, 178, 185
head injury, 159, 162, 170, 176–8
healthcare
  practice, 110–13
  regulators, 17
Health Education England, 24–5
heart attacks, 27, 74, 101, 152, 172–3
  see also myocardial infarction
heart rate, 71, 149
hernias, 76, 188
heuristics, 49, 56–61, 126fig, 135, 153, 199
Hierarchy of Competence (Maslow), 139
high blood pressure *see* blood, pressure
hindsight bias, 74, 167
history taking, 42, 51, 55
Hitler's sweater, 79
holistic acumen, 15
HPC (history of presenting complaint), 167–8, 172, 176, 181, 185, 189, 192
human error, 69, 120, 173
  see also errors
human factors, 20, 61, 69, 77, 79, 88, 94, 114, 120, 169, 171, 173, 177, 178, 182, 186, 191, 193
human fallibility, 70–71
Hume, David, 52
humility, 47, 61, 74–5, 82–3, 90–1, 120–1, 124t, 197
Huxley, Aldous, 74
hypertension, 172
hyperventilation, 168–9
hypoglycaemia, 38, 52–3, 76, 160
hypotheses and solutions line, 144fig
hypotheses, 56, 74, 112–13, 115–16, 119, 135, 142–6, 150, 158, 160, 170, 174, 179–80, 183–4, 187, 194
hypothetico-deduction, 49, 55–6, 58, 114–15, 125, 130, 160
  see also deductive reasoning

I

ideation, 72
if in doubt, don't, 55, 77
illness, 8, 11, 25, 29, 31, 42, 69, 99t, 111, 113, 154, 170, 173–4, 180–85
  see also case studies
illusory superiority, 139
imaging, 170–71, 190–91
inclusion, 81, 83, 88–9, 91
inclusive decision making, 81–105, 108
Indigenous populations
  knowledge, 83
  populations, 83–4, 91
inductive reasoning, 51–3, 53fig, 125
infallibility, 122
information processing, 107, 113–16, 143, 151, 169, 171, 173–4, 178, 182–3, 187, 193
informed consent, 42
in-groups, 85
innate egocentrism, 119t, 174
innate selfishness, 120t
innate self-validation, 119t, 179
innate sociocentrism, 119t
innate wish fulfilment, 119t
insight, 15, 45, 47, 61, 74–5, 83, 89, 92, 119–20, 137–140, 142–3, 139t, 171
  see also professional insight
Interpersonal Communication Competence Scale (ICCS), 98
interruptions, 62, 173
intoxication *see* alcohol
intra-cranial bleeds, 169, 171, 179
intuition, 40, 46, 58–60, 74, 76, 107, 114–16, 123t, 125, 134–5, 141, 143, 146, 149, 158, 173–4, 184, 191, 195
intuitionism, 28, 34, 41fig
intuitive responses, 168, 172, 177, 181, 186, 190, 192, 199
Inuit, 91
ischaemic bowel, 76

J

judgement, 2, 20, 35, 46, 58, 72, 78, 83–5, 109, 116, 122, 126, 133, 135–136, 140–2, 162
just culture approach, 45, 49, 61, 67–8

justice, 28–30, 36–7, 39, 41, 43, 47, 67–8, 73, 75, 152, 171, 184, 194

K

Kahneman, Daniel, 50, 56–8, 71–3, 75, 92, 107
Kantian autonomy, 31–2
Kant, Immanuel, 6, 28, 30, 32–3, 42
Keogh, Professor Sir Bruce, 7

L

language, 81, 91, 94–7, 99t
latent errors, 182
learning cultures, 68–9
learning disabilities, 185–9
Left in Care of (LICO), 156
The Linda Problem, 72, 75
logical intuition, 59–60
lone working, 169
long-term conditions (LTCs), 8, 11, 23
loss aversion, 73
LTCs (long-term conditions), 8, 11, 23

M

management, 9fig
Maslow, Abraham, 138–9, 161
Marshall, Albert (Elder), 82–3
means to an end, 6, 33, 42–3, 179
Mehrabian, Albert, 96
memory, 65, 69, 117, 139
mental capacity, 99t, 122
mental health, 7–8, 25, 47, 101, 160
mentoring, reciprocal, 93
metacognition, 92
Métis, 91
migraine, 168–70
minor head injury, 176
mistakes, 45, 49, 64–6, 65fig, 68, 70
Montgomery Rule, 33
multi-morbidity, 11, 152
Mumps and rubella (MMR), 108–9
myocardial infarction, 52–4, 74, 173, 175, 199
  see also cardiac arrest; heart attacks

N

narrow-mindedness, 124t
National Competency Framework for Paramedics (NCFP), 3–4, 7, 82, 91
naturalistic decision making, 49, 60–61
NCFP *see* National Competency Framework for Paramedics
NEWS score, 183
National Occupational Competency Profile (NOCP), 3
NOACs (novel anticoagulant drugs), 12, 177–8
no blame cultures, 69
noise, 43, 94, 182
non-maleficence, 428, 30, 35–6, 39, 152, 171, 184, 194
normative decision theory, 50
novel anticoagulant drugs (NOACs), 12, 177–8

O

omission bias, 77
omissions, 19, 46, 64–5, 69–70, 77
onward plan of care (Plan), 168, 172, 177, 181, 186, 190, 192
optimism, 73
organizational policy, 18, 65, 158, 164
outcome/hindsight bias, 74, 167
out-groups, 85, 93
overconfidence bias, 75, 190, 193
over-testing, 150–2, 158, 166

P

PAC *see* Paramedic Association of Canada
PCC *see* Paramedic Chiefs of Canada
PACE model, 163
pain, 29, 42, 100, 143
  see also abdominal pain; chest, pain
paralinguistic, 95–6
Paramedic Association of Canada, 2, 3, 33
Paramedic Chiefs of Canada, 3
paramedic ethical decision-making model, 40–1, 41fig
paramedic ethical model, 39
paramedics
  being ally, 88–9, 89fig
  career development, 4–8
  changing roles, 1–8
  cultural competency to cultural humility, 90–91
  curriculum, 2, 7, 12, 88
  diversity, encouraging, 92–3
  education and training, 5, 7–8, 23–4, 26, 88, 91, 178
  evolving role of, 1, 6
  literally, 25
  management, 8fig
  metacognition, 92
  professional conduct and standards, 5, 15, 20–22
  psychological safety, 68, 91, 97
  reciprocal mentoring, 93
  research, 8fig
  term, 1
  thought process, 92

unconscious bias, identifying, 87
unconscious bias training, 88
patients
ageing population, 13
data, 43–4
demography and epidemiology, 8
patient-centered care, 12, 15, 17, 29, 33, 42–3, 130, 175
safety, 46, 61–5, 67
pattern recognition, 49, 56
Paul, Richard, 118
peer pressure, 124t
peer review, 45, 153
performance, 2, 17, 62, 65, 78, 158, 196
personal values, 122
pessimism, 73
polypharmacy, 11, 152
population, 13, 143, 147, 151, 163, 199
see also demography
positionality, xv, 82, 84
positivism, 116
post-positivist, 116
pPCI (primary percutaneous coronary intervention), 173, 1751
pregnancy, 101, 115–16, 129, 185–9, 199
presumed consent, 42
pride, 122, 124t, 171, 180
primary percutaneous coronary intervention (pPCI), 173, 175
principlism, 30–31, 34, 36, 40, 47
probability, 73, 115
neglect of, 182, 190
pre- and post-test, 147, 150
procedural sedation and analgesia, 18–19
productive cough, 74, 142, 172–3, 181
professional identity, 7, 15, 20, 24–5, 46
professional insight, 15, 37, 45, 47, 75, 170–1, 174, 179–80, 183, 187–8, 190, 194
see also insight
professionalism, 5–7, 15, 20, 22, 43, 47
professional regulation *see* regulation
protected titles, 7, 17–18
psychological safety, 68, 91, 97
pulse, 71, 73, 76, 130, 149, 173, 182

Q

quasi-rationality, 134–5

R

reasonable alternatives, 33
reciprocal mentoring, 93
registration, 17–18, 120, 158
regulation, 1, 4–5, 15, 17–22, 43, 47
respiratory illness, 180–85
respiratory rate, 149t, 181
resuscitation, 25, 29, 38, 60, 63, 78, 130, 142, 169, 182, 194
see also CPR (Cardiopulmonary Resuscitation)
Return of Spontaneous Circulation (ROSC), 77, 173
ROSC *see* Return of Spontaneous Circulation
Royal College of Paramedics (UK), 23, 88
rules of thumb, 56–7

S

safe care, 82, 153–4
safeguarding, 28, 143, 187–8
safety, 46, 61–5, 67
Safety Netting, 49, 133, 155–6, 159–60, 163, 165–6, 169, 171
sanctions, 17, 19–20, 44
Scope of practice, 6, 18–19, 23, 171, 183, 197
secondary care, 163, 187
SEIPS (systems engineering initiative in patient safety), 64, 64fig, 67, 69
self-care, 11, 181
selfishness, innate, 120t
self-validation, innate, 119t, 179
sense-making, 133, 141–3
sepsis, 159, 175, 182–5
sexual health, 186, 189
SH (social history), 167–8, 172, 176, 181, 185, 190, 192
Shannon-Weaver model, 94–5
shared decision making, 33, 42, 145, 160, 195
shot-gunning, 126fig
sickle cell crisis, 101
sickle cell disease, 101
skills gaps, 186
smoking, 29, 54, 123t, 142
social media, 43–4, 108–9
sociocentricity, 119t, 121, 124t
Socratic Paradox, 138t
solutions line, 144fig
Specialist/Advanced Paramedics in Critical Care, 24
standards, 1–3, 5–6, 13, 15, 17–18, 20, 25–6, 46–7, 67, 91, 166, 175, 197
Stanford University experiment, 109
statistical process control, 78
STEMI care bundle, 175
stereotyping, 90, 125t, 173
stress, 20, 69, 110, 158
striking off, 123, 157
stroke, 37–8, 53, 76, 159
structured communication, 49, 69–70
ST segment elevation, 152, 175, 199
surgical errors, 70

suturing, 44
Syed, Matthew, 117
System 1 thinking, 58–9, 92
System 2 thinking, 58–9
system safety and reliability, 63
systems engineering initiative in patient safety (SEIPS), 64, 64fig

T

tacit knowledge, 60, 115
task-cycle time, 164
Tenerife air disaster, 74, 120, 163
terminations, 185, 187
thought experiments, 27
thought process, 92
training, 5, 7–8, 20, 23–4, 26, 51, 88, 91, 161, 178
Truth and Reconciliation Commission of Canada, 82, 91
Two-Eyed Seeing, 82, 83
Tversky, A., 50, 73, 75
typicality, of situation, 126fig

U

uncertainty, 59, 123t, 126, 143, 145, 163
unconscious bias, 86–8
  identifying, 87
  training, 88
unconscious competence, 139t
unconscious incompetence, 45, 139t
urinary tract infections, 23, 53, 186
utilitarianism, 27–8

V

vaccine sceptics, 108
values, 5, 20, 26, 29, 31, 71, 90, 107–8, 110, 113, 122
values-based decision making, 107, 110, 113
verbal communication, 95–6, 98
vigilance, 67, 151, 173, 182
violations, 64–5, 65fig, 67
viral infection, 111
virtue ethics, 30
vocabulary, 95
vulnerability, 171, 186

W

warfarin, 177–9
weakness, 53, 173–4, 181
WHO Surgical Checklist, 70, 121
wish fulfilment, innate, 119t
wishful thinking, 122, 125t
worsening care advice (WCA), 156, 159, 166
wound care, 176–7, 179
written communication, 97

Z

Zimbardo, Philip G., 109–10

Other Titles of Interest

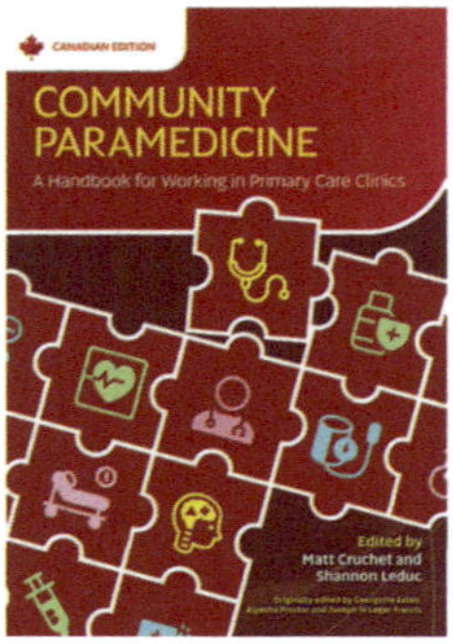

Community Paramedicine

Matt Cruchet, Shannon Leduc, Georgette Eaton, Alyesha Proctor and Joseph St Leger-Francis

ISBN: 9781801612210

Written by over 20 experienced clinicians, this essential clinical reference outlines the core skills for community paramedics working in primary care in Canada. Covering assessment, diagnosis, management, professional issues and real-world case studies, it supports both practising and aspiring community paramedics, with content fully adapted to Canadian practice.

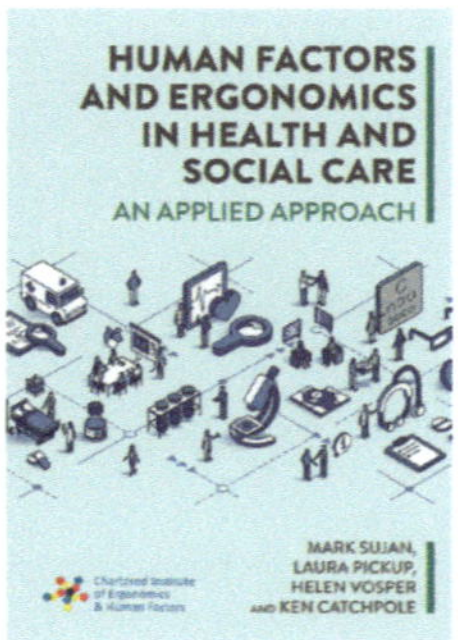

Human Factors and Ergonomics in Health and Social Care

Mark Sujan, Laura Pickup, Helen Vosper and Ken Catchpole

ISBN: 9781801610933

This practical introduction explains how human factors and ergonomics improve patient safety, staff wellbeing, and care quality. Using real-world case studies and system-based insights, it supports healthcare professionals implementing or applying human factors principles in everyday practice.

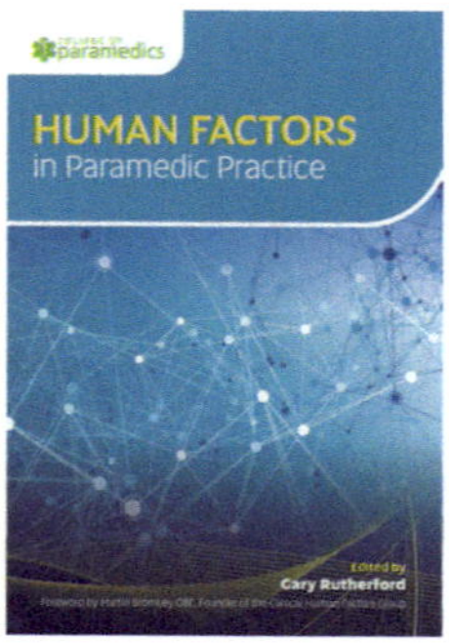

Human Factors in Paramedic Practice

Gary Rutherford

ISBN: 9781801610124

Designed for paramedics, this introduction to human factors explores the complex systems shaping pre-hospital care. Through real-world examples and systems thinking, it supports safer practice, effective teamwork and a stronger safety culture across paramedic roles.